Anointed
but SICK

OUR JOURNEY TO HEALING

Dr. Juanita Woodson

Copyright © 2018 by Dr. Juanita Woodson

All rights reserved. This book or any portion thereof may not be reproduced or used in any manner whatsoever without the express written permission of the publisher except for the use of brief quotations in a book review.

ISBN - 978-0-578-42498-9

Printed in the United States of America

First Printing, 2018

Impact Development Publishing

950 Eagles Landing Pkwy
Suite #722
Stockbridge GA, 30281

www.DrJuanitaWoodson.com

Table of Contents

Chapter One: I Need Help Jesus! 5
Lenika Scott

Chapter Two: The Spiritual Mind Over My
EARTHY MATTER 23
Tonya Joyner-Scott

Chapter Three: Broken But Not Destroyed 37
Melissa Osman

Chapter Four: I Am The Mustard Seed 55
Carmen Myrick

Chapter Five: I Can Do All Things Through Christ
Which Strenthens 67
Antoniia Perkins

Chapter Six: This Baby Will Live And Not Die 75
Lakeisha Martin

Chapter Seven: Anointed And Depressed 89
Ikisha Cross

Chapter Eight: Escaping Toxicity 101
Suprena Hickman

Chapter Nine: Sick, Going In Cirlces 117
Trisché Duckworth

Chapter Ten: Even In The Midst 129
Michelle Tutt

Foreword

On January 2, 2018, I found myself in a situation I never thought I would find myself. One minute I was making breakfast and the next minute I was sprawled across the floor at the base of the stairs having a heart attack right in front of my small children. My heart started racing, my palms got sweaty and I began to feel dizzy and light-headed, and apparently had fainted.

My husband had already left for work and it is by the grace of God that my oldest son, 10, had the wherewithal to quickly run to my bedroom, find my cell and call his dad. It just so happened that my husband was not loudly blasting his music in the car, and could hear his phone ringing. It also just so happened that he hadn't gotten too far from the house. Moreover, our neighborhood was a walking distance to the nearest hospital. Won't God order your steps?

Prior to my heart attack I had recently lost a considerable amount of body fat through working out and hitting the gym on a regular basis-and opting for a healthier diet. The thing that makes this book so relevant for me is that my health journey, Fierce to Formidable, was very public.

I had written books, workbooks, audios, masterminds, branded a t-shirt line and even launched a free support group for women that had close to 2,000 women in it. How could this be happening—now? And why? What were my followers going to think? Would this undermine my movement? Would it make women doubt my kingdom assignment? I had all kinds of questions for God. Why would He bring me this far to leave me and have me looking crazy for all to witness?

Fast-forward, after connecting with Dr. Juanita Woodson, a prolific teacher, trainer and prophetess, whom I have watched minister to and impact hundreds of thousands. I am all the more convinced of the power of our testimonies and how my sickness made me more anointed and not less. Having overcome so many adversities herself, and to see the anointing on her life, Dr. Woodson is undoubtedly the one called to usher in understanding around this topic. Why is this so important? Because we fear what we don't understand, and until fear is moved out of the way, we will not operate in the fullness of our power here on earth.

If we're not careful while we are in the valley, we will begin to doubt the anointing on our lives—even doubt our purpose and our will to live will come into question, despite a track record of wins! The testimonials and accounts in Anointed But Sick will show you the multiplicity of ways in which you can be on the top of the mountain in some areas of your life while suffering in the deepest valley in other areas. It will also illuminate for you that the sharpening of your anointing is taking place right under your nose.

I am convinced that living your best life requires owning your fierce, and that requires unabashedly operating in your anointing.

Dr. Shekina Farr Moore

Founder, B2F Girls | www.B2Fgirls.org
CEO, Intercontinental Coaching Institute | www.traintocoach.com

Introduction

In early 2016 I was headed home from an amazing dinner with my family. We had eaten at one of my favorite places and I was certainly stuffed. Suddenly I been to feel dizzy and nauseated, I actually thought I would faint at any moment. Soon after I began to feel my chest tighten and my heart started to beat extremely fast. I asked my husband to take me to the hospital because I was feeling sick. Immediately I remembered what my doctor had told me weeks before. I reached into my purse and pulled out a baby aspirin and took it. The doctor had warned me that if didn't watch my cholesterol she would put me on pills. She also told me that I was 1 point from being a diabetic and that if I didn't lose weight I would be on insulin medication. As my heart stopped pounding, I allowed myself to come to grips with the truth. I was too fat and I had to do something about it! I was 213lbs at the time, 5'4, and completely obese.

How in the world did I let this happen to me knowing that my mother and sister both died of the same disease? I literally watched my sister being butchered at the age of 42 as the doctors were trying to find a suitable vein to perform her dialysis. When they finally found a vein, the holes they dug in her leg would not heal. She began to decay and they continued to remove pieces of her leg until the entire leg was gone. She died from that infection. My mother started having strokes back to back shortly after my sister's death and died as a result. We were clearly dealing with a generational curse and it didn't care that they were both ministers of the gospel of Jesus Christ! Both had led countless souls to Christ through preaching and teaching in many churches.

I began to seek God on how to break this curse, live a healthy lifestyle, and lose weight in the process. As I searched and searched I found much information on how your blood type can directly affect your diet. Essentially, if you eat according to your biological make up, you will not have as many health issues and concerns. Not only did I study my blood type but I also studied how insulin effects fat production. It was ultimately determined that eating less meat, less sugar and less processed foods causes you to have better overall health. As I embarked on this God led journey, I have lost over 35 pounds and still counting. All health threats have ended. My sickness was obesity and a poor diet. What could your sickness be? Allow these women to pour into you faith from their stories of being sick but yet anointed. God has the final say and it is His good pleasure to prosper you in health even as your soul prospers! John 3:1-2 Beloved, I wish above all things that thou mayest prosper and be in health, even as thy soul prospereth.

I could tell you about several illnesses I have experienced over the years, but what is more important is the fact that God has delivered me out of them all! From Depression, ADHD, obesity, diabetes, high cholesterol, anxiety, and anemia, God has delivered me from them all! Be prepared to laugh with us and cry with us as we embark on a journey together to examine the truth behind being "Anointed But Sick".

Dr. Juanita Woodson
CEO- Impact Development Foundation
www.drjuanitawoodson.com

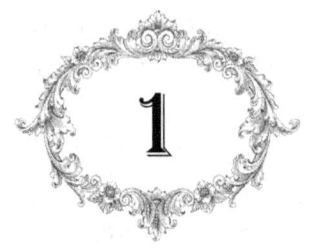

Chapter One

I NEED HELP JESUS!

Lenika Scott

I noticed I was quickly spiraling out of control as I found myself taking care of my husband, my 6 beautiful daughters, my extended family, my business and my ministry. I was Losing my grip and losing it very fast. A few short months prior, life was good. In fact VERY GOOD! The breakthrough I had been seeking and searching for years manifested and had knocked on my door. Many of the prophetic words, visions and prayers had found their way right to my path. My husband and I were traveling all over the world. Santorini Greece, Rome Italy, Venice Italy, Cancun, British Virgin Islands, South Africa, Dubai just to name a few. Our life was upgraded as we moved into our beautiful home paid for in cash, yes totally debt free which had always been a dream of ours. We found ourselves doing things we had longed for, for so long. Please allow me to take you back in time for a few minutes.

You see when I got married I married very young meeting my husband and at the tender age of 18. We quickly started a family and life as we knew took us on journeys unexpected. We had to learn the art of shifting and maneuvering and shifting and moving very fast. As I pursued my career God had another plan and when you say YES to your will Lord, the reality looks very different than what you (think) He has in store. I'm sure you can agree about that! Instead of being a career and working woman I found myself behind the four walls of my home as a stay at home mom growing a beautiful and strong relationship with Jesus and also learning the art of prayer and fasting. Holy Spirit started revealing my purpose and the plans he had for me. During which time, He drew my heart toward desiring a home based business and creating wealth from home. Though it now look as though it happened overnight that couldn't be furthest from the truth. The years of learning, growing, building, adjusting and readjusting were so needed for the weight of success that would come ultimately our way.

You ask, what does this have to do with you being anointed and sick? I'm so glad you asked.

Like many women who put themselves on the back burner feeling like they have to save the world, I was that person. I was the person who would tarry with you for an hour in prayer until I felt heaven move and a release take place. I was the person who would try to be there for every single person that needed my attention yet still run a household and business at the same time. Yeah right? I know I may sound a little sarcastic sisters but no one will be able to push and push and push without something being sacrificed in return and for me it was my health. At first it was breathing problems and chest pains. I found myself in the emergency room and the hospital for tests and next thing you know they are running cat scans and doing MRI's to do cross checks trying to get the root of the problem. I would leave the emergency room or the doctor office come home, rest for a little and the next day I would be back up pushing again. Inwardly saying to myself, "I will be okay"!

I remember at one point and time my husband and I hired a personal trainer and while I was in a session I almost passed out. After experiencing this a second time we decided something more was going on so I removed myself from training for a short time. A few doctors' visits in between but there was no hard-core diagnosis, so I continued doing the same things. Then we decided to see another trainer who worked in the area of light work training and after a few visits with me he asked me, "do you have Fibromyalgia?" What? "Fibromyalgia, the devil is a liar"! Yes sad to admit, that was my response. He then went on to mind his business but he couldn't help but notice the areas that he would help stretch me would be areas of noted pain for those who have been diagnosed with fibromyalgia.

Well.... the minor and very light training became too much for me. On some days, I could barely get through a 30 minute session without pain or shortness of breath. I had to withdraw from those sessions.

I found myself quickly going downhill in a way where it seemed as though I was losing my grip. The sickness was interfering with my everyday life. The normal things such as cooking, cleaning, laundry speaking on the phone became a challenge. I found myself in bed day in and day out. My body was wrecked in pain and I wasn't aware of what was happening to me. I begin to seek the Lord for answers and one day I was led to google signs of Fibromyalgia and my mouth dropped. Wait a minute? Not me! This can't be true.

In front of my eyes I was reading "Fibro Symptoms" and each and every symptom, yes you got, I was experiencing.

Widespread Pain
Neck pain, back pain, shoulder pain, hip pain, leg pain
Fatigue
Sleep Issues
Brain Fog
Depression and Anxiety
Irritable Bowel Syndrome

After going to google I realize that I had just about every symptom and then came the "pain point test". It is a test where doctors check areas of your body for pain and if your body is sensitive to touch in those areas fibro may be the cause. Sure enough after visiting the doctor to have them verify what I already pretty much knew, the doctor gave me a diagnosis.

Mrs. Scott, you have fibromyalgia!

Though I'd already figured that was the case and this was in fact what I had been dealing with long before even speculating, the weight of the diagnosis became so unbearable to me within that first 24 hours. My body started flaring up like crazy just with the news. I was in so much pain in my back that it felt like someone was placing a hot iron on my back and my shoulder blades.

So now what Lord? What do I do? I have so much to do! I have kingdom work.

For a few days, I took the medication the doctors prescribed but when I started walking around like I was a zombie I knew this wasn't my destiny. I told myself I'd rather be in pain and try to function than be in pain yet have no recollection of what was happening around me. With the mediation she prescribed I felt as though I was there but I was away somewhere. My thoughts were I can' t operate like this.

Frustration set in. I found myself angry and upset and then repenting for feeling angry and upset. I was experiencing heavenly encounters on one hand and terrible pain and turmoil on the other hand. There was a serious battle going on and as days progressed I found myself sinking into depression. Battles in my mind were strong. Questions coming from my soul but the most asked question was...

Why me Lord? The answers would be returned void, Or so I thought!

So I found myself beginning to push in the midst of the pain still thinking that I was superwomen. This lasted only for a few short months. Let me explain. I would get on my prayer call but prior to getting on to minister it took everything in me to press. The whole time I would be making myself to the bathroom to face my face and brush my teeth I would be praying, Lord give me strength, I am hurting and my body is in so much pain. Help me push through Lord! Some mornings getting up I could barely walk. By His grace I would make myself downstairs to my prayer room to go live for prayer. Some days I had to hold on to the bed, furniture or to the wall to help me get from point a to point b.

During the time I was dealing with all of this, my prayer ministry had been going forth for 10 years surely I couldn't let

God down and the people down. (Just letting you know my thoughts). When we would travel, my husband would be so protective of me even to the point of him taking me out of our meetings and our events early that I may go back to the room to lay down and rest. When we would fly into different states it was no site seeing, enjoying ourselves or none of that but flying in heading straight to the room for rest.

Strange thing about it was this, from the outside looking in know no one knew I was sick. I massed it very well especially on social media. Due to the following and my business connections via online sure enough I can't let them know what was going on with. Of course those who were close to me knew something was going on. One days my baby sister called and said, "Nik you look so sick, your eyes have dark circles around them." Of course I ended up having to share with my following some of what I was going through and you will read about how I got help very shortly as I had to pull away and take a 2 week sabbatical. So for months after being diagnosed, trying to hide it, still trying to move as normal I hit ROCK BOTTOM!

Yes! I hit ROCK BOTTOM! With my anointed self.

One day while being in my prayer room and to be honest I had become a little disgusted with my situation. When you have the will and drive to accomplish goals, to soar high, to do the will of the Lord but your body doesn't to want to cooperate it becomes challenging. I was in my prayer room and such a sovereign act took place as I cried out to God.

I said, Lord "I NEED HELP"!!!

Then they cried to the LORD in their trouble, And He brought them out of their distresses. He caused the storm to be still, So that the waves of the sea were hushed. Then they were glad because they were quiet, So He guided them to their desired haven. Psalm 107:28-30

Therefore let us draw near with confidence to the throne of grace, so that we may receive mercy and find grace to help in time of need. Hebrews 4:16

And it seemed like something literally broke for me in the spirit realm. Something truly happens when you cry out to God from a pure place of surrender. And a few short days thereafter a holistic doctor by the name of Dr. Roni came into my life and boy did she change my life. I found out she had a holistic clinic where her specialty of critical care was in the area of treating patients with Cancer, Fibromyalgia and Lyme Disease.

When I found out that Fibromyalgia was critical my thoughts were wow, only your grace dear Lord! We discovered it was considered critical because it is a "whole body" condition.

I took a HOLISTIC approach to receiving healing!

We set up an appointment, and my husband and I went to her retreat clinic which was in Martha's Vineyard and we participated in her 21 day detox program. Our total visit on the island were 14 days however we continued to program for 7 more days after our departure. I say we because my husband decided to go forth with the program as a support. So as I went through this medical detox I learned so much about my body and my health. I also learned God had been trying to get my attention for a long time.

After running blood work it was reveled that my adrenals were OUT. Not only was I diagnosed with Fibromyalgia, I also had adrenal fatigue. Commonly found in individuals who push themselves far beyond what is normal. It is when your body is in fight mode all the time.

And my body was saying ENOUGH! I don't like how you have been treating me and I am shutting down!

People who experience fibromyalgia also have high levels of stress and have a high level of inflammation in the body. Since the stress hormone cortisol is also a natural anti-inflammatory, having an adrenal system that is working overtime can actually raise those cortisol levels too high and block your immune responses.

My body was so toxic and it was screaming at me! My first day there, I instantly went into a healing crisis. After only a few hours of detoxing I got very sick as the toxins were finding their way into my blood stream. My husband was concerned and asked the doctor, what's is going on with her? And she calmly said "she is in a healing crisis". Your wife is very toxic and anytime a person detox, when the toxins that are in the organs and gut get into the blood stream they feel it and they feel horrible. Yes day 1 my body was responding due to all of the sickness and disease that had found its way there. Speaking of sickness and disease I remember around the third day we had to do a coffee enema. I know it sounds gross my husband jokingly now calls it a coffee enemy but I must say they work like magic! During the first one, I actually smelled sickness leaving my body. This was problem one of the strangest things experienced while there. Something totally unexplainable but it was what it was. I smelled sickness and disease leaving my body. Very emotional experience to think all of that was inside of me.

During another detoxing session which was a colonics I literally saw BLACK STUFF leaving my body. While laying on the treatment table tears begin to fall down my face. All I could do was think, I am sick, I've been so sick and I didn't realize the magnitude. My body was literally the breeding ground for cancer and although I cringe at the writing of that word the irony is, it was so!

Basically in short detoxing the body brings the acidic body to an alkaline state. Sickness and disease doesn't like a body that is alkaline.

So as I begin to detox and go through natural treatment I learned so much and one of the things I learned and I am so certain many Christian women have found themselves in this same place. I wasn't taken good care of my body. I could pray and prophesy the house down, tap into the spirit realm where the supernatural release would take place but again I wasn't doing right by my body.

What? know ye not that your body is the temple of the Holy Ghost which is in you, which ye have of God, and ye are not your own? 1 Corinthians 6:19

Our doctor taught us the importance of herbs and natural healing and though we've heard these things for years, the level of awareness was astounding. Personal awareness is actually a dangerous thing, When a person is aware they can do some serious damage to the kingdom of darkness.

And on the banks, on both sides of the river, there will grow all kinds of trees for food. Their leaves will not wither, nor their fruit fail, but they will bear fresh fruit every month, because the water for them flows from the sanctuary. Their fruit will be for food, and their leaves for healing." Ezekiel 47:12

I will share some of the herbs they used during the detox program for those of you who are reading this and my story is moving you because you feel as though the Lord is leading you to a holistic approach.

The Lord used Apostle Juanita as she released a prophetic word to me regarding helping many women who were suffering in silence with sickness and pain. She said God is calling you to teach his daughters about health, healing, wholeness and taking better care of themselves. She saw a vision and another platform released and also said God has allowed you to go through this for a greater witness!

Beloved, I wish above all things that thou mayest prosper and be in health, even as thy soul prospereth. 3 John 2

God revealed to me that He could have healed me SUPERNATURALLY, but if he healed me and I went on to do the same things I was doing before it would have been null and void and the sickness would have returned.

My days consisted of a daily protein shake which included mixed berries, 2 live green drinks, a power packed vegetable soup for dinner. In a typical day, you will drink 40-48 ounces of water, 32-40 ounces of herbal tea, 16 ounces of vegetable-based soup, and 32 ounces of either a green drink made from vegetables, vegetable juice, or a berry drink. Below is a list of some of the foods and some natural holistic treatments you can do at home

Ozone Water Daily	Sweet Potato
Bone broth	Beets
Turmeric	Mint
Lemon	Parsley
Cucumbers	Cilantro

Ginger	Coconut
Kale	Coconut Milk for smoothies
Celery	Minerals and Vitamins
Strawberries	Lymphatic Massage
Blueberries	Body wrap in sauna (removing toxins)
Rasberries	Colonics
Garlic	
Coffee Enemas	

MANY different essential oils were used
It was like a method, feed the cells flush the toxins.
Nutrients in and toxins out.
The good in and the bad out.
Detoxing Tips
Switch out all sweetened beverages
Only water or herbal teas
Stay well hydrated
No sugar during the detox
Think Green (The more green the more alkaline)
No processed or refined foods
Raw veggies and Raw fruits
Walk 30 mins a day
Rest well 8 hours of sleep
Minimize sleep
List of Detox Foods

Spinach/Kale: These leafy greens are both great sources of amino acids (protein), calcium, beta carotene (vitamin A), vitamin K, iron, manganese, magnesium, zinc, folate, and selenium. All around super foods, spinach and kale are great for strengthening the body, creating beautiful skin, boosting the immune system, and providing important antioxidants. Also, each is full of fiber which is great for cleansing the colon!

Cucumber: Highly hydrating, cucumbers are full of B vitamins, silica, and electrolytes that help build clearer, brighter skin. The vitamin C, caffeic acid, and electrolytes in cucumbers makes them great at fighting puffiness and bloating in the body, working as an anti-inflammatory team.

Celery: Very alkaline, full of calcium, magnesium, and potassium. Good source of B1, B2, B6, and C vitamins, folate, iron, and amino acids. Celery helps to lower high blood pressure and reduce puffiness. It contains compounds polyacetylene and pthalides which reduce inflammation and stress (causing blood vessels to dilate), respectively. Celery is a powerful detoxifier and colon cleanser.

Pear: Contains vitamins C, E, B, and K, copper, manganese, potassium, iron, magnesium, selenium, calcium, zinc, and folate. Pears are wonderful for the skin and supportive of both the lungs and the colon.

Lemon: Extremely alkaline, are high in vitamin C, and traces of calcium, potassium, and magnesium. Lemons are a powerful detoxifying agent. They support liver function, purify the blood, destroy free radicals and toxins, flush out bacteria, fight wrinkles and rejuvenate skin. Great for long-term weight loss.

Chia Seeds: These seeds swell 10 to 15 times their original size when placed in liquid, which makes them great for weight-loss. They also help stabilize blood sugar levels, providing you with longer lasting energy. Chia seeds are an excellent source of protein, calcium, anti-oxidants, and omega-3 fatty acids.

Mint: Great source of vitamin C and beta carotene (vitamin A), copper, iron, potassium, magnesium, and calcium. Mint aids in digestion, is helpful in relieving congestion of the respiratory tract, and lowers blood pressure.

Parsley: A powerful detoxifier, parsley aids digestion, removes toxins from the body, acts as a diuretic by flushing out the kidneys, and purifies the blood. It contains vitamin A, C, and E, folate, iron, and anti-oxidants.

Cinnamon: Studies have found that cinnamon helps lower blood sugar, have anti-oxidant effects, fight bacteria, and reduce inflammation.

Ginger: Helps ease nausea, maintain proper blood circulation, improve nutrient absorption in the body, is anti-inflammatory, strengthens immune system, and fights common respiratory problems.

Turmeric: Very high in anti-oxidants, turmeric is a great anti-cancer agent. It is also anti-inflammatory and works as a blood cleanser. Cleansed blood results in clearer, brighter skin.

Cayenne Pepper: An incredibly potent spice, cayenne pepper is often used to detoxify and cleanse the body (mostly due to capsaicin). It has anti-cold/flu properties, aids in digestion, has anti-fungal properties, helps discourage formation of blood clots, supports weight-loss, promotes heart health, and aids in joint-pain relief.

Detox Smoothies

<u>Green Protein Detox Smoothie</u>

- ½ cup unsweetened almond milk

- 1 tablespoon almond butter
- 1 banana
- 2 cups mixed greens (kale, chard or spinach)

Glowing Green Detox Smoothie

- 1 kiwi
- 1 banana
- ¼ cup pineapple
- 2 celery stalks
- 2 cups spinach
- 1 cup water

Apple Berry Detox Smoothie

- 1 cup mixed berries (like raspberries, strawberries, and blueberries)
- 1 large apple
- 2 cups spinach
- 1 cup water (or unsweetened almond milk)

Pineapple Banana Detox Smoothie

- 1 cup pineapple
- 1 banana
- 1 apple
- 2 cups spinach
- 1 cup water

How am I doing now? I am on the road to recovery! Not 100 % out of the woods but definitely not where I was. Recently we had to return to the island for a metal detox and I got very emotional as we were walking through the airport. This time I could walk at a good pace and not have to worry about stopping every other minute. While there at the retreat I kept thinking the Lord that our visit 'felt' so different. My thoughts were, "I feel good"! Things were different the last time we were here.

To my beautiful sisters in Christ!

Hopefully my story have helped you and if God has been dealing with you about taking better care of yourself please heed his instructions because the Father always knows what's best.

Prophetess Lenika Scott

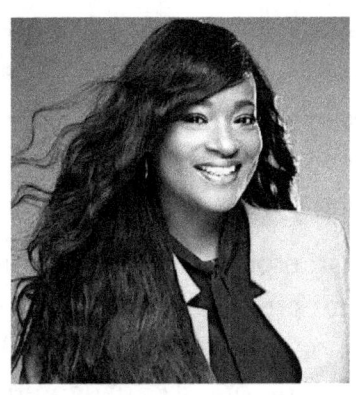

Lenika Scott Ministry Bio

Lenika Scott, a woman of strength, love, and integrity, is the epitome of the Proverbs 31 Woman... "She looketh well to the ways of her household, and eateth not the bread of idleness. Her children arise up and call her blessed; her husband also and he praiseth her. Many daughters have done virtuously, but thou excellest them all." (Proverbs 31:27-29)

And excelled, she has.

Her vision and insight are like no other. Pure heart and clean hands. She is a prophetess, intercessor and worshipper. A true child of The King, whom he uses to set the captives free. She has been chosen because of her passion for healing and deliverance to those in bondage, crossing boundaries to see this accomplished. When going into battle, it is an honor to have her on your side. The anointing and mantle that she carries is one of a knight. A Royal Knight of The Kings Table.

In 2009, God opened the Heavens over Lenika's life. She experienced a major breakthrough in business after partaking in a 21 Day Fast.

He then shared with her that many Christians needed to understand the power of fasting and how fasting with prayer can break open many things that are being held back. This ultimately led to Lenika Scott releasing her first book, "Fasting for Breakthrough" how a 21 day fast can change your life.

Lenika is a marketplace minister, multi-level marketing guru, life coach, entrepreneur, successful businesswoman and mentor. With guidance and help from God, she manages an immaculate household of six daughters while being a submissive wife to her wonderful husband Gregg Scott. With dedication to her self-worth, she strives daily to keep herself healthy, fit and lovely.

In 2007 she was a mom who decided to leave her career to stay at home and give her children a more stable, loving environment. It was a financial sacrifice to give up her salary of over $50,000. However, she and her husband agreed that the needs of their children outweighed the pursuit of her career. Lenika was always ambitious! She decided to turn to the Direct Sales industry to earn extra income from home and contribute to the bottom line of her family's financial state. This decision would be one of the most pivotal decisions of her life. As she looks back, she realizes and admits this was a spirit led decision.

God is raising her up during this season to teach his people about wealth, debt freedom and living a victories life. Not only in the area of spiritual healing and deliverance but also finances. God has allowed her and her husband to break many records in the business arena but most importantly they both have been very instrumental in helping others break free financially.

She is a voice for this generation and a force to be reckoned with.

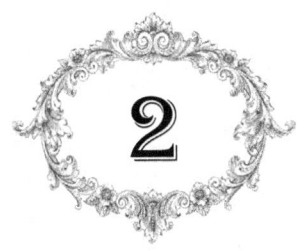

Chapter Two

THE SPIRITUAL MIND OVER MY EARTHY MATTER

Tonya Joyner-Scott

Barren: not producing or incapable of producing offspring; sterile: a barren woman. Unproductive; unfruitful

The definition of a Proverbs 31 Virtuous Woman didn't include any words like sterile, unproductive, unfruitful or being incapable, but that is what was spoken to me as I sat in the examination room with my husband and listened to the report from our doctor. Can you imagine how I felt in that very moment?

Do me a favor and allow me to take you back a few years prior to this moment. I am a widow. For two years my late husband and I tried to conceive a child. We wanted three, four, or even five children! We already had one beautiful daughter, but oh boy we wanted more! Well, what's the problem? I'm cycling every month. I must be ovulating. Every month I would pull out my calendar and count one, two, three..., fourteen, fifteen, sixteen and find my ovulation period. When those days came around, let's go!! Let's make this baby! But nothing happened. It's funny, there was a time before we were married when I was waiting anxiously for my period to come on, because we didn't want to pop up pregnant. I mean what would people say? What would my parents do? Later I found myself waiting anxiously for it to NOT come on, because we wanted so desperately to have a child. Month after month, there it was again. Another HEAVY cycle that lasted 7-10 days every single month.

We finally decided to see a doctor. They are now trying to determine what the problem could be. We were asked to come back another morning, but prior to us coming we were instructed to be intimate. They wanted to test him and see if he was still able to produce a child. Well, we arise bright and early and followed our doctor's orders, arriving on time to our appointment. I prepare for the examination as we wait patiently for the doctor and nurse to arrive. I tell you, it's funny, they're testing him to see if he can still produce a child, but I'm the one on the table. When you think about it, it's really a beautiful honor to be a woman. We're the receiver. We're the carrier. We nurture his seed, so if it wasn't him, they would then know it was something wrong with me.

The examination is done, and we waited patiently for his return. I can still remember it like it was yesterday; his words exactly. "He can populate the world! We don't want him to, but he can." We laugh in agreement, and he then looks at me and says, "This means it's you. And we're gonna have to find out what's wrong."

I can remember thinking in that moment that this must be why I never conceived a child as we dated. He asked me to marry him in 1993, and soon after that, I conceived BEFORE the marriage took place. If you didn't know, I'm a recovering people pleaser. The type of person who never wanted to make mistakes or disappoint others. And then, right here as everything seems to be turning out picture perfect, (for a people pleaser) I go and get pregnant! Like my granddaddy would say in that good ole southern kind of way, "Got to be mo' careful!"

We had a beautiful baby girl, got married and was ready to have more, more, more! But all of that soon came to an end as in the months to follow, we learned he had an aggressive form of brain cancer. My life had suddenly changed. I now stood as a twenty-nine-year-old widow, holding the hand of our 5-year-old little girl. It's clear to see that having children was no longer on my mind. I was simply in survival mode.

One day while driving home I passed a gentleman working in his yard and we wave to each other. He was on the phone with a friend of his who also knew me. His friend was actually my loan officer who had also supported me by purchasing dinner plates from me and my family while my husband was fighting cancer, and he also helped us move into a house from the apartment we lived in. As I drive by, he tells his friend, that I had just passed by and asked if he knew how I was doing. This friend decides to call and check on me after they hang up and immediately I knew who it was. I recognized his voice. It was so good to hear from him as he had truly been a blessing to our family. I considered Dexter Scott, a really good friend.

As the conversation was coming to an end I suggested we meet up for dinner maybe? Here's the thing, when I said it, I was just thinking I would be catching up with a friend of the family. He, on the other hand, heard something different. I know that now, but I didn't know that then.

The evening we got together for dinner was fun and filled with great conversation. While sitting there he's also having a conversation with God. God is telling him that I am his wife to be. Yes, while I'm eating chicken wings, he and the Lord are over there discussing our future together. Turns out, He was right!

We fell in love, got married and yes, we wanted children. I was ready immediately because I was already over 30 years old. My heart's desire was for my daughter to have siblings growing up with her. So, guess what? Suddenly, what that doctor said to me a few years prior is now in the forefront of my mind, again. I remembered that the doctor had turned to me and told me that my late husband could populate the world. Our not being able to have a child is because something was wrong with me, but I never found out what that "something" was. That was one of the toughest conversations I had to have with my husband. He is such a family man. He comes from a large family and they are very close. They grew up with cousins upon cousins and every holiday is always filled with fun, laughter and excitement! Being a husband and a daddy are two of the most important titles and responsibilities to my husband. This is truly an honor for him and he puts his wife and his children at the top of his list. As we try to conceive a child in the first year of our marriage I'm back to counting again: one, two, three…, fourteen, fifteen, sixteen; its ovulation time! But, nothing. Year two, still nothing. In the third year of our marriage, we decided to see the doctor. Testing Dexter wasn't necessary; we already knew it was me. They ran a few tests and did some imaging of my reproductive system. Now, let's come back to that moment that he and I anxiously waited for the report from our doctor.

We all know how it is when things look and feel different when you're nervous. We weren't doing too much talking as we were simply waiting to hear what the doctors had found. The door opens and my husband stands and comes to stand beside me as the doctor comes in and takes his seat. He has images of the photos taken of my ovaries, fallopian tubes and uterus. He explains to us what everything is. My husband stands there with such a stern look on his face as he stares at the screen and listens intently. His right arm is folded across his chest as his left elbow rests gently on his hand while his thumb and index finger cup the left side of his cheek and chin. The doctor then tells us, "You won't ever have children because your ovaries are twisted and your fallopian tubes are blocked." He then goes on to say, "At least you've had one child." In that moment, tears began to roll down my face. Dexter still has that stern look on his face. He glances over at me and sees the tears and shakes his head very sternly at me "NO" and points UP! His hand never leaves his face. Immediately I take a deep breath in; I wipe the tears away and come into agreement with my husband! In the deep breath I took, I simply thought, BUT GOD! The doctors told us one thing, but we made a decision in that moment to TRUST God and take Him at His Word!

Who can relate? You can hear the world's facts, but our charge as children of God is to trust His Truths! The facts were my ovaries were twisted and my tubes were blocked. Well how did this happen? Throughout my teenage and young adult years I had cysts on my ovaries and fibroid tumors would develop in my uterus, my tubes and I had very heavy menstrual cycles. I'm thinking that this may have been the cause, but honestly, no one has ever said. But, the TRUTH is...God's Word says.....

As another year passed and we're still believing, I must admit, my faith began to dwindle. All around me other sisters were having children. Right here in the Scott family, my brother and sister in law were having one beautiful baby girl after another! And here we sat, nothing, one month after another; one year after another, nothing. I felt worthless. I hated that I could not give my husband a child. I even questioned God as to why would He give Dexter a wife that couldn't give him children? Although he already had a child from his first marriage, being able to see his daughter and spend time with her the way he desired was painfully limited. I repeat, it was painfully limited. And now here he is married to me and my reproductive system is no longer reproducing.

I can remember crying out to God one evening as I laid in bed cramping and bleeding. I found myself feeling so depressed as my menstrual cycle was back again. Honestly, I began to think I was being punished for being intimate with my husband before we married. You see, when Dexter and I started dating, this was the first time I dated anyone as a born-again Believer in Christ. I began to think that my reproductive system was locked up because I did not wait for my wedding night to give myself to my husband. Here I am, a child of God, yet unable to have children. I must have done something wrong. Here we are praying and believing God for a child and one month after another, no pregnancy.

I know, I know..., God isn't vindictive, but the attacks on my mind were severe and this is what I was thinking. I found out years prior that something was apparently wrong with me but, here I am thinking that I am being punished for what he and I had done prior to our getting married. This is what caused my faith to dwindle. I didn't talk about it, but I carried this with me day after day after day. My mind wasn't on what I wanted, but instead on what I didn't want, yet I'm looking to conceive. The enemy attacks our minds in an attempt to weaken our weapon of warfare... our faith. You produce in your life what you think about, be it good or bad. Your thoughts are your beliefs and your expectations come from these thoughts. I wanted a baby, but I thought more about not having a child than I did about having this bundle of joy. I thought more about reasons why this isn't happening than I did about what it was going to be like feeling this miracle move around inside of my womb. Here I am trying to conceive a child with a mindset of being barren. I was receiving what I was "truly" believing for. Transformation happens from a renewed mind. I needed to renew my mind.

In the days to follow I received a word from a male co-worker with instruction for me and my husband. He told me that my husband and I needed to go on a 9-day fast and trust God for the birth of a child. Wow! God sent this African man to me, out of the blue, with instructions to fast and pray about the birth of our child! This Word and these instructions did something to us and our faith! We obeyed and started the fast right away. This is when the renewal of the mind started. My expectations changed. Dexter and I told God we believed Him, and we took Him at His Word.

Faith without works is what? You got it, dead! My once dead faith was now alive and in the book of James, the scriptures to follow tell us that our faith is shown by what we do. This resonated with me majorly so, one evening, in the middle of the night we decided to demonstrate our faith. We got up, got dressed and drove to a 24-hour Wal-Mart to purchase a baby's diaper bag. We told God we believed Him for 2 babies, so guess how many diaper bags we purchased? You guessed it, two! We didn't care what the doctor's said. We took God at His Word and trusted Him! Our faith was ignited to be fruitful and to multiply!

Our language changed. The extra bedroom in the house was identified as the nursery, the baby's room. If there was something to take to that room, we would say, "Put this in the baby's room." Or, "Take this to the nursery." My renewed mind brought about a transformation for me. It felt so good and I could truly feel the difference in my state of being.

During that time, my sister in law was pregnant with their fourth child and we continued to rejoice with them for conceiving and having another precious baby girl. No matter where you find yourself in life, rejoicing with others is so important! Others may not be dealing with what you are, and the devil would have you feeling jealous and envious. This produces strife, disorder and all kinds of evil. He would want you thinking on those things, rather than on what is honorable, just, pure, lovely, and commendable. God teaches us if there is any excellence; if there is anything worthy of praise, we should think about these things. This is the power of your mind and your thoughts becoming things. This is your transformation happening from a renewed mind. Your faith is your substance and your evidence of what you are believing God for, and it won't be weakened. Remember, the enemy wants your mind. He wants your thoughts. He wants to weaken and/or destroy your faith. Don't let him.

We continued to live our lives with high expectation. I could see the baby in the nursery and looked forward to purchasing the crib and decorating the baby's room. We would even look in the backseat, visualizing and imagining the baby safely strapped in the car seat. It was fun and always brought joy into our hearts and minds. In essence, we begin to think on what we wanted, not on what we didn't want. In other words, I stopped thinking about not being able to have a child but thinking about our life with our child.

The peace of God was truly surpassing our understanding. So much so that I didn't realize that we were at day...twenty-nine, thirty, thirty-one, thirty-two, thirty-three... Wait a minute! Dexter! Let's go to CVS! My energy level was through the roof! And so was his. We jumped in the car and took a 5-minute ride to what was a 10-minute norm. Those automatic doors opened and without thought, we headed down the aisle that we had grown so familiar with. My heart rate was pounding as I was nervous and excited all at the same time. I mean, what if I'm not? Do you know how many times I took a pregnancy test only to have my cycle come on the next day? But this time, I'm at day thirty-three. Could this be my miracle?

We arrive home and I head straight to the bathroom to take the test. Guess what? I didn't have to wait 5 minutes to see the 2 blue strips appear. They appeared immediately! I tested positive and, in that moment, we praised God for the miracle of life He had placed inside of me with my twisted ovaries and blocked fallopian tubes. Dexter and Tonya Scott were pregnant!

Is it going to be a boy? Is it going to be a girl? We really didn't care, but a boy would be awesome because Dexter and his 3 siblings all had girls. His oldest sister Dawn had 1 girl, his brother Gregg had 4 (at the time, they now have 6), and his sister Hope had 2 girls. He marries me, and I bring my little girl and remember Dexter also had a little girl when we married. It would be nice to have a little boy, but I was so happy to be pregnant, I really didn't care. On January 6, 2006, we birthed Morgan Kennedy, another beautiful Scott baby girl. Morgan was a beautiful blessing from God and we were so grateful to Him for the birth of our child.

Morgan took her first steps at 7 months. It blew our minds that she started to walk at 7 months. I remember someone saying to us that she was getting out of the way for another child to come. We laughed as we knew that I still had blocked fallopian tubes and twisted ovaries. We were thankful for Morgan and honestly, we weren't thinking about having another child. We had Tailiah, Kiera and Morgan and were satisfied.

I can still remember the day I came home from work and I was so tired. It was a different kind of tired and was very unfamiliar to me. I also felt nauseous. I just needed to rest so I curled up on the couch, work clothes and all. In the coming minutes it hit me! My eyes popped wide open. I gasped and then sat straight up! I wondered, "Am I pregnant?" I drove to CVS and purchased a pregnancy test. Guess what? Dexter and Tonya were pregnant again! All I could think about was when we purchased those two diaper bags that night in Wal-Mart. We told God we believed Him for two babies, and He did just that. Here I am pregnant again, before Morgan even turned 1 year old. On July 12, 2007, we gave birth to Tyler Alexander. Yes, you got it, the first grandson to Dexter's Mom & Dad and the first nephew to his siblings.

Born to me, the woman who felt worthless.

Born to me, the woman who thought she was being punished.

Born to me, the woman whose faith was shaken.

Born to me, the woman who came to her senses, as a child of the Most High God, who took Him at His Word and changed her thinking and language. I believed Him. Dexter and I did exactly what he motioned for us to do that day when the doctor told us that we would never have children and those tears started down my face. Dexter looked at me with a stern face and shook his head "No" and pointed his finger "UP" to the Heavens. I dried up those tears, we came into agreement and started through our process.

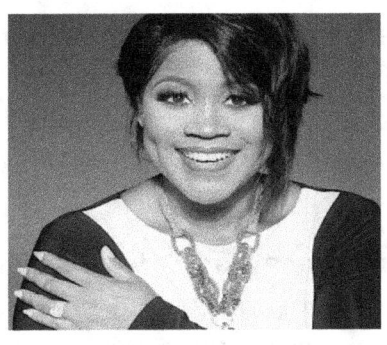

Tonya Joyner-Scott-Bio

Inspirational

Tonya Joyner-Scott has spent years motivating and inspiring audiences to get out of their own way and take a front-row-seat in life. Her reputation as a gifted and inspirational speaker, trainer, and spirit-driven success mentor is spreading throughout the business and faith-based community. Her trainings are impacting thousands of individuals who seek financial growth, emotional restoration, and spiritual transformation.

Conversationalist/Speaker

It is more than just speaking; it is a conversation! Sometimes you just need someone to talk you through the process of getting to the next level in your life. Tonya is pointing her audiences to pursue their passions through honest dialogue that leaves them ready to run to their personal finish lines!

A Certified NBC University Speaker, Tonya draws her strength from her faith in God and her personal experiences.

Pulling from life-lessons learned from personal trials and tribulations, Tonya Joyner-Scott brings forth engaging and stimulating presentations using candid examples and sharing stories that her audiences are able to connect with and draw from.

Tonya has an uncanny knack for immediately captivating your thoughts with her serious yet pleasant demeanor as she strives to get key success nuggets to you. The best you lies somewhere within, so when Tonya Joyner-Scott speaks it forces you to tap in to that undiscovered GREAT YOU in order to fulfill your divine destiny and accomplish your vision.

Mindset Coach

What you focus on the longest becomes the strongest. Tonya and her husband have been fascinated with the mind and how it operates for years. A Certified Coach with SRT Global, she and her husband are a part of a global mission to help people to completely reprogram their mind, remove any mental and emotional blockages or stop patterns from their past, so they can Create the Life they were meant to be living.

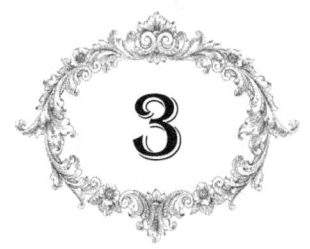

Chapter Three

BROKEN BUT NOT DESTROYED

Melissa Osman

This is my personal story of struggling with depression, anger, anxiety and more while holding on to my faith and love for God and believing in a better day. At ten years old I was removed from my adoptive home and put into a hospital due to me having a nervous breakdown and attempting suicide after I felt there was no other option or way out of my abusive home life. Every cry had gone unheard. I could no longer go back to the torment that I was enduring. After being released from being hospitalized I spent the remainder of my childhood in group homes and Foster care. After a few failed placements in different facilities and a foster home I was transferred to Youth Villages in the winter of 1994. While in Youth Villages I spent many years waiting in a group home for either a foster home or a family to adopt me. I continued to struggle with myself further while I watched other girls meet their families and leave while I was left to wait. I wondered what could be so wrong with me that no one wanted me and couldn't understand why?.

The one thing that remained stable and kept me was my Faith and Love for God. At the age of thirteen my mentor whom I called Mom was assigned to me through Youth Villages. Before my Mentor was introduced to me they warned her how broken, difficult and damaged I was. My mentor still took on the challenge any way. I struggled with myself, depression, loneliness and feeling as if I didn't belong. As a young child dealing with physical and sexual abuse as well as losing everyone I loved, I hated myself. I hated even looking in the mirror. In dealing with all of these emotions and issues within myself I became angry. As a result of the overwhelming emotions and anger I began to mutilate myself punishing myself to try to ease the pain. To some these behaviors such as self-mutilation and suicidal attempts may be crazy. However to the person dealing with the overwhelming emotions and pain, it is real. I prayed and asked God to take my anger so I wouldn't be bitter. I spent a lot of years being angry. I still talked to God and I prayed daily. I was still dealing with enough anger, depression and anxiety that Youth Villages felt it was necessary to put me on twelve different medications.

The medications were only quieting the storm still raging within me instead of resolving the real issues at hand. I remained in the Youth Villages while waiting on a foster home for three long years. During those three years my Mentor spent a lot of time with me and treated me as her own child. Our bond quickly grew. She had a difference of opinion about me needing the medication that was only drugging me. My Mentors family was the sweetest people who never judged me, was stable and never made me feel out of place. I was at home when I was with them. I never wanted to go back to the cottage at Youth Villages. We did everything a mother and daughter would do together. Things I had never been able to experience before without restraint like shopping, eating out, swimming, taking walks, cooking, decorating the house and more. To me it was the simplest gestures that mattered most. I asked my Mentor and her husband if they would please adopt me. Due to my mentor and her husband's extremely busy schedule as well as demanding lifestyle they did not feel like they could parent me. Again I was crushed. I was beginning to feel like the Dr. Seuss bird walking around asking, "Are you my Mother"? The one thing that my mentor gave me that impacted my life more than anything was unconditional love. No matter what I did or how I did it my mentor never stopped loving me no matter how difficult I was.

That was the best medicine a kid could have. During the three years that I was a resident at the Youth villages Cottages in Tennessee I had bonded close to several staff members. As fast as the staff would come in they would leave out. This just created further instability and abandonment issues for me causing me to become more hopeless and depressed. Eventually there was a staff member that I bonded very close to and I respected her very much. As often as the staff member was able she would take me off campus to her family's home always making me feel safe at home and loved as well. My staff member and her husband requested to adopt me however it was denied due to the staff members personal involvement as a staff member at Youth Villages. Again I was crushed. Unlike the rest of the staff members I did remain in contact with her. We began calling each other sister as we are only about 10 years apart and extremely close. After three long years waiting for a Foster home a door was opened. I was allowed to go to stay a weekend to decide if I was compatible with the family or not. Despite all hesitations due to realizing the family had many issues that were going to be challenging, I decided to go because it beat being stuck where I was. I was moved from the Youth Villages Cottage to the Foster Home within a few days. What was challenging quickly became unbearable in the home.

Due to my Foster family things escalated where my counselor moved me to another Foster Home in another County. I had a Foster Mom and a Foster Dad who were both teachers. They took very good care of me, helped me in my schooling, pursuing my writing career, being active in church, fixing me up a bike and my own room and they gave me that unconditional love. I had a very close relationship with God and my prayer life was extremely important to me. I was learning to Love myself and focus more on my strengths verses my imperfections. After all the happiness, achievements and love unfortunately there was still this huge void in my life. "My mother" I wanted and yearned for a relationship with her. At the age of 17 I began searching for my biological Mom and a year later I opted out of states custody. Holding onto every promise she made to my Foster parents and myself I packed up everything that I owned and with a little U-Haul behind my Moms vehicle I went to live with her. In the beginning everything was a little difficult but it was manageable.

My Mother did not seem to be able to communicate very well with me and our relationship quickly became strained. I bonded with my Step Father and he was extremely supportive towards me even taking on a second job to help support me while helping me through school. He was my rock. One night while gathering work uniforms from my dad's vehicle I severely injured my foot and lower leg due to hurricane winds. After many weeks of seeing specialist as well as receiving MRIs my diagnoses was that I had torn out all of my ligaments, nerves tendons and did further damage. I wasn't able to walk and I was not getting any circulation to my foot or leg at all. I had to be braced, casted and put on complete rest staying off of my foot. I had to learn to walk again receiving many treatments, shots, physical therapy and more. The stresses and strain of trying to catch up with my credits that were altered from moving from another state were difficult as my classes were extremely advanced. Also going to school while in severe pain and receiving all of the rigorous treatment took a toll on me. I began to relapse suffering from depression resulting in severe migraines. I eventually had to be home schooled. Although my mother quite her job to take me to my appointments there still seemed to be a disconnection between us. Every attempt I made to bond with my mom failed. It only further hurt me and angered me. I regretted leaving my life I had with my Foster Family but I realized it was too late.

    I attempted to contact them however due to an inability to reach them I figured they must have retired and moved. The unresolvable issues between my Mom and I caused my depression to become so extreme I no longer desired to eat, drink, or even be involved in anything. While I lived with my Mother I kept in contact with my mentor. My mentor paid for a ticket for me to fly and see her. During my vacation to visit her we got an urgent phone call that caused me to end my vacation and quickly go back to my Moms house. My Step father had suffered a massive stroke but was persistent in requesting to see me. As my Mom picked me up at the airport from flying back I knew nothing was good any more after she made it clear to me that she no longer wanted me there with them. It wasn't long after I graduated from High School that my Mother put me out in the middle of a lighting storm resulting in me living with my neighbors.

While living with my neighbors I worked at a nearby hotel to pay for my bus fair to go back to Tennessee and I attended summer school to obtain a higher diploma. After working and saving up I caught a bus back to Tennessee. My mentor was waiting at the bus stop to pick me up and all my possessions that I could carry in 2 foot lockers. It was the best feeling to be back with my mentor. I lived with my Mentor for a short amount of time while Youth Villages was preparing me to go into a brand new program called assisted living for adults who outgrew the system with nowhere to live. I worked with my mentor to find an apartment. Youth Villages assisted me in furnishing my apartment as well as the first months bills while I looked for a job which didn't take long. I quickly obtained a job, was promoted to manager and I began paying my own bills. I enjoyed being an independent adult, handling my own responsibilities and living on my own but I was lonely.

Due to pet policies my Mentor and Youth Villages owners wife found me a kitty I named Angel who helped me through a lot of hard times. Later I met a guy whom at my young age I felt that I was in love with. The instability of everyone in and out of my life and the issues with my Mom created a huge void for me. The more I hung out with this guy the more rebellious I became and the further I pulled away from everyone else including my mentor. He showed me all the signs that he was no good but I was used to men treating me that way. I felt if I loved him enough then he would stop being abusive. I blamed myself for the abuse thinking I just needed to do better. I had all the ignorant thoughts that young insecure and troubled adults have. I eventually allowed him to move me out of my apartment and into his home. The abuse got worse. My crazy thoughts of reasoning and finding excuses for his violent behaviors and lies seemed to be endless. Eventually this led to me barely waking up in the hospital to identify myself as well as my bloody clothing to the police. I stayed there for many days while I recuperated from him trying to kill me, leaving me for dead in a field. When I left the hospital I was transferred to an abused Women's shelter and then went into homeless shelters. I began putting in many applications for jobs. I eventually landed myself a job at the local Kroger Grocery store. Being in constant survival mode I stayed exhausted and I began struggling with anxiety. Some nights I slept behind dumpsters.

During those stays at these shelters I met a really nice man who loved God and was in charge of serving the lunch food at the church. My faith was at an all-time high as once before in my life and nothing was going to stop me. He showed me the word and claimed that God said I was his wife. Proverbs 18: 2-24 "A man who findeth a wife findeth a good thing, and obtaineth favor of the Most High" It was the word of God so it has to be real right? After many weeks of us being homeless on the streets and spending time together we decided to get a rooming house together and then a house that we paid for through remodeling it. After getting married to meet the requirements of living in a church home and obtaining jobs we decided we wanted a baby. As I kept other people's children, became a Sunday School Teacher, a Vacation Bible School Teacher, a Tutor and Mentor to other children I still felt an enormous void. There was still a deep yearning for a child of my own despite what the doctors said about me not being able to conceive. Knowing the odds were against us we cried out and prayed for our miracle child. Things began to change in our home. My husband rarely came home. When he did he was extremely violent.

So I prayed. One night he came home and passed out in the floor I demanded him to give me answers because he was barely able to wake up. My worst fear was real. What he told me was lies and what everyone else was telling me was the truth, he finally admitted to being on drugs. I no longer prayed for a child, I cried out to God to deliver me from the toxic situation. There was no way I wanted to bring a child in this world into a situation like that. Through prayer and Faith I maintained my sanity while continuing to endure violent attacks from him. We had no electricity, food or money. His job didn't exist and he took my money that I earned. When he came home he would beat me raw with metal hangers until I blead and solid metal rods to where I was unable to walk. Nine months after being clear from my ovarian cancer I found out that I indeed was pregnant.

So many emotions flooded me. I knew whatever happened I had to protect my baby. At 18 weeks after a brutal attack from him I found the courage and strength to escape my Domestic Violence situation. I moved in with my Mentor until we found a multiple roommate rental. One out of four of the room mates had 2 dogs whom she felt that it was acceptable to allow them to use the bathroom all over the house and destroy it to the point it wasn't livable. After several request to have the situation cleaned up and sanitized I had to move out. I had no other option than to move out for the safety and well fare of my unborn baby. My main focus was my son and providing for him. My sister continued to help me out a lot also helping me get my apartment together during the early stages of my labor before my son was born. As the 17th hour of labor came and complications became worse from the nurses giving me too much epidural my Sister rushed to be by my side during my final stages of my delivery. I could not even feel to push so my sister had to coach me on how to and when to push. My whole entire pregnancy all I could think about was all the fun things we were going to do together just me and my little boy.

As I got ready to leave not being able to stand up or move without severe pain continued. I had to leave my baby in the hospital another night due to his jaundice although they released me. I cried the whole way home. During the next 4 weeks I adjusted into being a Mama. My son was an amazing baby. I was overwhelmed with joy but unexpectedly depressed too. I worried I couldn't be the Mama I needed to be and I tried to get every detail of caring for him correct. He was born full term with premature lungs and esophagus. Caring for him was a challenge as he would constantly stop breathing and strangled on his formula every time I attempted to feed him. He required different breathing machines, breathing treatment tubes, air purifiers as well as monitors that had to be with us at all times to keep him stabilized. After just getting settled and in a routine my world suddenly flipped upside down. I woke up in the hospital where my sister worked at.

They were attempting to take my newborn son. It was difficult for me to speak or move although that was irrelevant at the moment. With my weakest voice I told them, "You want my breath then you take my son". "You want my son you take my breath". I had just suffered a stroke one month after giving birth to my son. As the days moved forward it seemed like I lived in the hospital with my son clinging to life. I never left his side even though the nurses begged me to go home. I crawled in the bed with him holding him and caring for him around the clock. It was very emotional and difficult for me. My son was an exceptional baby. He was my motivation. I rehabilitated my own self gaining strength in my legs by walking while holding on to his stroller and lifting cans daily for exercise. My goal was to be able to throw a ball to him by his first birthday. He was extremely smart and talking in short sentences before the age of one. He was advanced in everything.

He was a fighter and my world. During one of our trips back to our home after a few months of not being involved with my ex-boyfriend he held us against our will at gun point following us back to our apartment. He continued for months to physically abuse me causing many injuries and even rupturing my eardrum. My son and I broke free after we were able to get to the doctor by telling him I received a letter that my cancer was back. We were checked out and released to a Women's Shelter. While at the Women's shelter I was told that we could not be allowed to stay given the history of the abuser. They told me that I was putting everyone else at risk being there. With little to no options they contacted my biological Mom and asked her to come get me before he killed us. My Mom and Step Father did come and helped me get what they could hold in their van mainly of my sons belongings and we took off. From the beginning my mom informed me that the only reason why she came to get me was the ladies at work warned her that it would be her fault if she didn't come get me and something happened. My Mom seemed to really love her grandson but the relationship between us was too difficult. I ended up being hospitalized from complications of injuries received while I was being held hostage. I could hear everything but I wasn't able to respond of my Mom speaking as if I was dead and never coming back. About a week later as I started coming back and I was able to speak I was moved into a room where I had a roommate. We talked discussing my situation and became friends.

The lady provided information to help me get my own apartment. It wasn't too long and I was out on my own just my son and I. We went to church and we were getting along well. It was extremely difficult trying to take care of my son and being on a walker restricted to movement, no feeling in my hands and continuing to have seizures with small TIAs. Through my doctor a nurse was referred to come in and help me in my home. My son's health continued to struggle and a lady from the church as well as my friend from the hospital helped assist me in caring for my infant son. Seven months after being perfectly content with being single I became involved with another man. I hadn't seen my son that happy in a long time laughing and lighting up. After time went by and we spent more time together he was also abusive. I refused to leave him because he was terminally ill and I became pregnant with our daughter.

I wanted our daughter to have her Dad in her life as much as possible, but that came at a cost. As our daughter turned four months old he continued to be unfaithful, lie, be abusive and I found pornography with animals and children on his computer. I was fed up, disgusted and horrified by the inappropriate videos and there content. I stayed up all night packing all his belongings and we immediately separated. Through all of this I continued to struggle with postpartum depression and trying to manage it. I reached out for help and received treatment in a hospital after every attempt to regulate me on medicines failed for one reason or another. I was doing pretty well with two very young children whom required all my attention all the time with little breaks and little to no help. I wouldn't have traded it for anything in the world. I loved being a Mom. Shortly after I became stabilized from my postpartum depression my daughters father felt he didn't have the control that he desired of me and the children.

He made a false report to children's services in order to gain custody of them. Children's services came in and picked me apart making false allegations and writing up a false report concerning me. He was not providing any support for the children. I was struggling although the children were happy, healthy and didn't want for anything. My son continued with severe mental health, behavioral issues setting fires, running away, destroying things, violent behaviors and more. He was unable to receive any professional help until he reached the age of four years old. I had an appointment set up as he was nearing the age of four. Until the appointment I had to deal with his behaviors as best as I was able. His behaviors were increasingly becoming worse and they were exhausting. A huge investigation was started that turned into many years of the children being moved in and out of the home without any investigations or probable cause to take them only threats. My daughters biological Father was finally arrested after many years that the state allowed the children to be abused by him and his male friends. After the death of my daughters father I fell on financial bad terms losing our home that my daughter and I lived in resulting in the permanent loss of my daughter due to becoming temporarily homeless. I got professional help by a domestic violence counselor after I lost my world and a huge chunk of my heart. I continue to struggle without my children. It is a huge void and injustice but I'm making much healthier decisions. I've recently remarried to a good man and have started to pursue my personal carrier and I am currently helping my husband with his own business ventures while enjoying the farm we live on together.

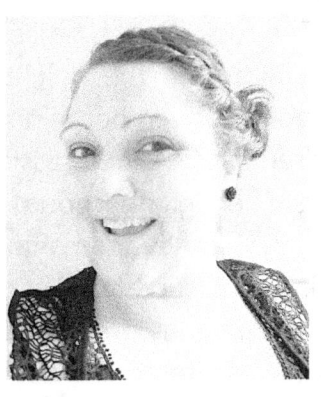

Melissa Osman Bio

Melissa Osman is an Author, Coauthor and Creative Artist. Since the young age of four her objective as well as long term goals have been centered on helping people, while also focusing on making a difference and impacting others' lives. She has a strong passion and love for others. Every opportunity she's had from the age of 10 to help a neighbor, friend or relative she's done so without complaint or rebuttal. Melissa began babysitting at the age of thirteen. She has obtained an extensive history of volunteer work and ministry. In Jackson Tennessee she volunteered in four different Elderly homes assisting in scheduling activities, birthday and holiday celebrations as well as individual care for those who did not have families to visit them. Melissa was a volunteer for habitat for humanity helping build houses for less fortunate families.

While living in Memphis Tennessee she spoke for Youth Villages a program for troubled youth. She assisted in the homeless ministry feeding them and handing out clothing to those in need. Melissa was also a Sunday school teacher, mentor, tutor and an event coordinator while assisting in children's ministry. She took it upon herself to gather toys and distribute them to children in the neighborhood. When she moved to Georgia she continued her ministry. She babysat the neighborhood children and helped assist the elderly with cooking and cleaning in her neighborhood. Melissa also assisted in the Church ministry where ever a hand was needed such as fund raisers, janitorial work, secretarial paper work and events. Whenever the opportunity was presented for Melissa to help someone she never has hesitated and has always found a way to support and assist people. She desires to continue in her ministry to impact and strengthen others during and after their struggles. She is working towards many future projects to protect the Youth, strengthen families and bond communities closer together.

At an early age Melissa had great Faith and love for God despite her situations and circumstances that seemed to be a night mare that she would never wake up from. As an infant she was adopted. She suffered from depression and anxiety partially as a result of being in an abusive environment until the age of 10, group homes and finally foster care. She had a difficult time with self-esteem due to abandonment issues, severe trauma, physical abuse, sexual abuse, isolation and constant instability. She often questioned her worth. She used to always question God why? Why would he allow her to go through so much hurt and pain? Into Melissa's adult hood her depression continued through more abuse, losses, toxic relationships, illnesses, lack of support and financial difficulties.

Despite all her efforts she also lost custody of both of her children after the system failed to protect them. She felt the most pain ever and truly didn't know how to move forward. Her kids were her life and world which her days revolved around. It was through her Faith that she drew every bit of strength to endure her trials. Every single loss and all her pain one thing remained the same. God's Love and Favor for Melissa. No matter what God never left her even if everyone else did. That strengthened Melissa and changed her perception on life; she began working on changing her negative mindset despite her trials beyond what she felt she could endure. At times she felt she might die in it. As Melissa began to change her mindset despite her current situation and circumstances her life began to change. Her depression decreased from her lack of negativity being released into the atmosphere.

There is power in your tongue as well as your thoughts. Proverbs 18:21 Death and life are in the power of the tongue: and they love it shall eat the fruit thereof. A boat will not sink because of the water around it. When the water enters in that's when the boat will become heavy and drowned. The same goes for the negativity around us can only impair us if we allow it to get inside us and weigh us down. Through the transformation of her thoughts, consistent prayer life as well as mirror therapy she has become stronger. It has given her the ability to focus on her strengths verses her weaknesses. She says we all have a day or a moment but we don't stay there or allow our minds to take vacations there. Only short trips and back to kingdom business. Melissa says reflecting is good because it allows her to see her personal transformation flourishing. She is growing where she is planted and staying dedicated to not only her changes but impacting others as well. She has made better choices and has begun pursuing her dreams and goals for her future. " Yesterdays the past, tomorrows the future, but today is a gift. That's why it is called the present". Written by: Bil Kean

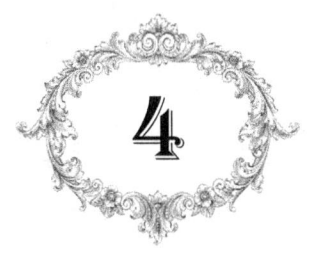

Chapter Four

I AM THE MUSTARD SEED

Carmen Myrick

"Had you not come in tonight, you would have died" words I've heard too many times to count over the last 8 years. For someone who has spent their entire life battling with their weight, I was blessed to have never encountered any sort of health issues. However, in February of 2011 that all changed.

I was in my second trimester of my 4th pregnancy, with my youngest daughter Camora. In general, this pregnancy was draining the life out of me. I was over 30 and much heavier than I was with my other 3 children. Nonetheless, I went in for my regular prenatal appointment and was experiencing excessive swelling, headaches, and seeing what I explained as little floating sparkles. It was no surprise that my doctor sent me straight to the hospital where I was diagnosed with preeclampsia and immediately admitted. My doctor ordered bed rest and wanted me to remain IN THE HOSPITAL until further notice. As a single mother with 3 other children (one being behaviorally challenged due to the trauma from my previous marriage), being on bed rest was already out of the question but staying in the hospital was not going to happen! Given the circumstances I ended up going home and attempting to give bed rest my best effort. This would be just the beginning of my fight with my health.

"God, why do I have to deal with this on top of EVERYTHING else I am dealing with?" Was constantly my question, "Ms. Myrick, please understand this is called the silent killer, so you need to be sure you're following my instruction" my doctor continued to tell me. I attempted to watch my diet, I exercised as much as my energy allowed, and I took my medications as prescribed. Did I mention how tired I was all the time? I literally would lay around like a vegetable praying for a supernatural miracle that would allow me to have enough energy to do anything beyond required life activities; working, taking care of my kids and my own basic needs. The fact was I felt worse, although my blood pressure was under control with the medication something within me was getting worse. Now how many know that as mothers, much less single mothers we do not tend to put ourselves first? That meant my personal solution to caring for myself when I felt sick was water, Tylenol, and a nap.

This I did for about a year until one day it seemed as if my whole life tried to shut down. That day I woke up late but was preparing for my good friend Trish to come in town for a visit. I literally could barely walk, I was exhausted with a headache and horrific cramps. I attempted to take a shower and became sick, throwing up blood and practically about to collapse. She just so happened to be arriving and she pulled me from the shower, got me dressed and took me to the hospital. I met an

ER doctor who sat with me and asked tons of questions, looked at each medication in my purse and tested me for everything imaginable. He then revealed that the hypertension specialist that I had been seeing all year had me on a bad combination of medications. This was of course making me sicker and after a series of tests I discovered I had kidney damage, poor liver function. and cardiomyopathy. This ER doctor recommended me to a doctor at the Sentara Heart Hospital in Norfolk, VA and adjusted my meds from about 5 different types to 2. Within two weeks I begin to feel less like a vegetable, energy increased, swelling decreased, and just began to feel more like myself.

I love sharing this story because of the supernatural element! I called back to the hospital to find out if this doctor worked out of a practice because I wanted a primary care physician that would be that caring and thorough. Crazy thing, no one had any clue who I was talking about. I had his name from the discharge paperwork, but no one knew the name. I asked if he was a nurse or a resident. I knew I was calling the right hospital because I always went to the same location, but just in case, I called all the Sentara hospitals in the area. Not one location knew of this man! You know what my conclusion was, clearly this doctor was an angel. I had no reason to believe otherwise, he was so kind, patient and attentive, but given the mystery surrounding his identity there was no other explanation. It was just a reminder of God's presence during my suffering.

When people talk about being sick we usually are referring to being sick in the physical sense. But what about the impact that sickness, stress and struggle have on our mental and emotional state? I found it hard to stay up many times because

I physically felt ill and it played on my emotional state as well. I struggled with depression and anxiety, my mental and my emotional state has often been a reflection of how I felt physically and with what is transpiring in my life. I was so concerned about how this was affecting me that I began to research different forms of depression. I quickly found out I was identified with situational depression, which is considered a short-term depression induced by stress of many forms. After experiencing a series of traumatic events this is considered a type of adjustment disorder. This can be triggered through grief, illness, relationship issues, work or school difficulties, financial problems, and numerous other adversities. But what if your life has been a constant and continuous cycle of all these things? Think about how the effects of those events come down on you after so many years.

My story doesn't necessarily end there, regarding the condition of my health. Fast forward to today, I am still fighting quite a few health issues, in addition to economic difficulties, family issues, career challenges, and so on. But, by God's grace I am still here. Through all my battles I have never lost hope that God's promises for my life would come to pass. He has shown me from the time I was a child His plan for my life and it is an amazing one full of joy, peace, and purpose. There have been times where I just laid on the floor crying out to Him because my life continuously manifested the opposite of the vision He gave me. Being that I am a fact and information driven person and tend to be very analytical, I would often question what God was saying and showing me. I am a who, what, when, where, and why kind of person. Does that make any sense? I hear what you are saying Lord and I see what you are revealing but my life does not add up to either in any way shape or form.

I need to know how this will happen; what do you want me to do; who do I need to be in relationship with; why are things so upside down all the time; what have I done wrong; how do I correct it; where do I need to be in terms of timing and location? I know that sounds crazy, but this is how my brain has been managing things for a very long time. When you feel like you have a history of messing things up and you are trying to course correct your life, this is the type of battle you deal with in the mind. I just wanted to make the right decisions and do the right things and feel my best while doing it.

For as long as I could remember, even when I was consulting God on things, I have had to make survival decisions: A decision to get me through what was occurring at that moment. So even in me thinking I am making the best decision for NOW it did not mean I was making the best decision for what lied ahead or long term. God will help you make momentary decisions that is true, but when the urgency in that situation is over your outcome will still be stuck in that right now decision you made. That is exactly what was happening with me. I was making sick decisions while in a sick state, making decisions based on the circumstances of now instead of destiny decisions and decisions based on God's will, plan and purpose for my life. I struggled with viewing myself as He showed me and only seeing where I was and how I felt.

I began to seek God for specific ways to cope with stress and trauma. After all, I did not have the time, insurance or money as a single mom to do counseling or buy meds; and until recently I did not make self-care a priority. God began to give me strategies for coping and revealing to me that self-care is MANDATORY. In terms of handling my own personal stress, God gave me a process that contained 3 steps; emotion, processing, and execution. I had to learn that an emotional reaction is completely normal, and I encouraged it. As a matter of fact, I found out that for me, God was encouraging it as well. The difference is how long do you stay in that emotion and what you do afterwards. The emotion part of my process allowed me to have that emotional reaction and depending on the circumstances I could be there for a few hours or a few days. Either way, I always allowed myself to feel it out, I cried, I slept, I retreated from life a little bit to deal with myself and how I felt about what happened or what was occurring. Processing, this is where I included the analytical part of who I am. The who, what, when, where, and why of what happened and how I got there. God is a huge part of this process because I am asking Him questions and seeking answers to make corrections not only within myself but if there need to be changes with anything around me that contributed to the problem. Finally, execution is where I am acting on what God has revealed. Taking steps to make changes or following the instruction on the things I need to do to basically level up from what has been happening in my life. These steps helped me to fight my depression and anxiety with His help and not add stress to my body that is already suffering from different illnesses.

Self-care is self-explanatory! Start taking care of yourself! I had to begin to give myself some attention. This has been a process because I am not in the habit of putting myself first in any way. I am still trying to perfect this behavior, as my illnesses and the medications keep me drained and I struggle to find the energy for much, but I am working on it! I made it a point to engage in more things like my quarterly spa visit for a facial and massage, v-steams (which are healthy by the way), detoxing, and of course my monthly hair and nail/pedicure appointments. I treat myself to small things when I can, accessories, books (I love to read) mugs, hats, journals, etc. little things that I love and can manage to afford on a regular basis. You would be surprised how just making those changes boost your spirits and put you in a better mindset to persevere through the days that you feel your worst or dealing with the most. It is ok to put yourself first, self-care is not selfish! God wants you to love on yourself, if not more than He wants you to love on others. I know we joke about cliché terms, but you cannot pour from an empty cup! Dealing with health issues takes a toll on your mind, body, emotions and spirit. He wants us in our best state of mind to be able to walk in our destinies and embrace His promises. Not caring for yourself and giving yourself proper attention will indeed lead to additional and unnecessary stress and depression.

Once you begin doing this you will be amazed at how your overall functionality improves. I am constantly reminded of God's love for me as even during illness, job loss, divorces (2), homelessness, relocations, emotional and physical abuse, a pregnant teen daughter, a son with emotional and behavioral disorders, one child with autism spectrum disorder, broken relationships, you name it and I have endured it. Only a God as amazing as He is could allow you to have ideas and multiple business ventures while going through all these things! Half of the time it seems as if my brain is hardly working because of the mental fatigue and physical exhaustion of infirmity and life challenges in general. However, He has still given me a level of creativity that has allowed me to start several businesses, a charitable foundation to help support other women, assist others in doing the same while being a mother to 4 children and a grandmother to my spunky little grandson. I can only gather that I am enduring so that on the other side of adversity when I reach my destination in where He wants me to be that my overcoming will be to help others overcome.

    I would never had gotten through any of these times without my faith; my personal relationship with God and my prayer life have been my lifelines. This is my personal journey and experience with illness, depression, and anxiety. I have made it with pretty much God alone and no therapy and medication; but by no means does this mean that you won't need either of the above. God has given me so much grace and blessed me with life despite carrying sickness for months, at times years were untreated because of my economic circumstances or not taking the time to even see about myself. Do not be afraid to go be seen by a physician, or to admit you need help, do not be afraid to be open with someone you can trust that can offer love and wisdom. To this day because my body is tired and in pain it attempts to dictate my emotions. I am more aware of it now so when it begins to happen I can correct it before it completely takes over. I spend a lot of time during the day just randomly talking to God because of how I am feeling physically and emotionally. It has been the only way that I have been able to maintain my sanity. I have not had therapy or support groups or even too many people that I on a consistent basis share my exact feelings with. When people ask, "how do you do it?", it is not a cliché answer to simply say GOD! Regardless, of what I have encountered, how depressed I may have been, or the times I was in tears because of anxiety, God pulled me through it. Having even only a glimmer of hope is all God needs to pull from to keep you on the right track. (Matthew 17:20 He replied, "Because you have so little faith.

Truly I tell you, if you have faith as small as a mustard seed, you can say to this mountain, move from here to there, and it will move. Nothing is impossible for you.")

    The one thing I am always certain of is His presence in my life. I have endured a lot of mental, emotional, and physical trauma, however, during all that God has continued to give me vision, ideas, and strategies not only for myself but for others. He has used me to help people get through their own personal battles with sickness, divorce, job loss, parenting dilemmas or whatever someone has needed me for. God always has made sure He has given me the words and wisdom that person needed at that moment. Despite my illnesses, despite my own emotional state from whatever I was dealing with at that time. It almost seemed as if helping others through their own personal storm while in my own became a form of therapy. It can be draining sometimes, but again, that is where that self-care comes into play and refueling spiritually on a regular basis and not just when I am empty. My family gives me purpose and a reason to keep going. My mother, has played a major and consistent role in my life making sure I am always reminded of who I am in Him and that I am smart, kind and beautiful! My children Cierra, Alicia, Aaron, and Camora have been my team and my biggest reason to keep going, along with my grandson Kaiden. We have endured many things, but one thing is for certain, they are built Ford tough like their mama and possess an even greater destiny than myself. I include my closest friends under the family umbrella because once you have walked a certain kind of journey with a person, sharing DNA doesn't matter. Your why is important, your support system matters, and God will deliver you from the hands of the enemy in health, career, finances, relationships and grant you the desires of your heart. What you want is important to Him, He just wants to be first and for you to never give up!

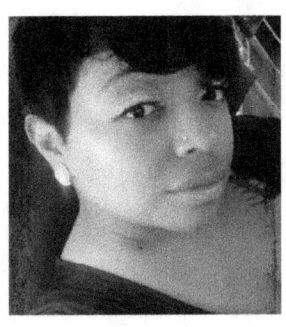

Carmen Myrick-Bio

Carmen Myrick is a woman of passion and purpose whose desire is to see others walk into their God given destiny. From a young age she was instinctively empowering and pouring into those around her. She is dedicated to see people healed and delivered from emotional trauma and live an authentic life of true fulfillment. Carmen has a heart for building women, specifically single mothers who want more out of life than what adversity they have faced and where it has left them. Additionally, young women who can be impacted at an earlier age before they encounter life changing decisions and situations. Her many years' experience as an entrepreneur, empowerment coach, mentor and advocate allow her to not only use the insight and wisdom she has gained through her own misfortunes and bad choices, but to see firsthand the brokenness that girls/women are in and create an environment of love and support to help them persevere through their own challenges.

As an entrepreneur Carmen uses business to mentor and empower those she encounters. Her love of beauty, fashion and business allows her to meet countless women who not only need her services and products but unbeknownst to them her God given wisdom and counsel. This has not only allowed her to service clients but minister to their heart and pour into their spirit and create friendships with people from not just other cities but internationally as well.

Carmen is the creator and founder of The Bella Boss Brand, LLC. a beauty, fashion and lifestyle company that works with small business owners to create magnetic brands that help position them to be the go to person in their industry. As a lash technician, she also created K'Moni Beauty, a lash & cosmetic company that celebrates universal beauty in all its' diversity. She is also the founder of HALO Charitable Foundation, an organization formed to be a support system for single mothers and women facing adversity. With her first love being music and called to ministry through creativity and dance, Carmen developed WOW (weapons of war) Outreach Ministries that ministers to the broken through the performing arts. Carmen is a writer and a serial creative who God has blessed with many gifts and abilities which she desires to use and give back to him by building His kingdom.

Though dealing with illness, trauma, extreme adversity, and just making many wrong choices Carmen has made it a point to honor God with her life by making a positive impact on others, even if only just one.

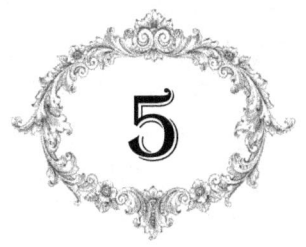

Chapter Five

I CAN DO ALL THINGS THROUGH CHRIST WHICH STRENTHENS ME
PHILLIPIANS 4:13

Antoniia Perkins

While growing up, I developed an active prayer life and I attended church services, with my family on Sunday's. As a child, I suffered from severe eczema, which limited my outdoor activities because my skin would itch and burn, when exposed to the sun. I was very sensitive to environmental stimulation, which entails, not being able to tolerate certain smells, noises and tastes. As a youth, I spent many days in the school nurse's office, with complaints of allergies, headaches, muscle spasms, various aches, pains and excruciating menstrual cramps (dysmenorrhea). I presented with the symptoms, of fibromyalgia. Conclusively, my diagnosis of fibromyalgia was about 20 years ago but I never allowed it, to stop me from accomplishing my goals.

I was an active member at The Rock Church, in Wilmington, N.C in 1999 (thru 2013). During my attendance at The Rock Church, I served in the infant room and on the intercessory prayer team. Although, the fibromyalgia would worsen, after the birth of each of my two children and I would remain fatigued daily with occasional flares. I was determined, to further my education. In 2005, I graduated from The University of North Carolina with a major in Criminal Justice and a minor in Theatre Arts.

In the summer of 2009, I suffered a horrendous fall, in which caused me to go into a fibromyalgia "flare." I also sprained my ankle and wrist and injured my neck, as well. This flare has lasted a considerably long time, in which all of my symptoms became exacerbated. Due to my injured neck (cervical muscles), I developed chronic migraine headaches. Chronic migraines are defined as, suffering from migraines for more than 15 days per month, over a three-month period. I can recall days where it was difficult to open my mouth or look at my cell phone because of the painful migraines. Before my accident, I was able to manage my symptoms well but after developing the chronic migraines, my life took an alternate route.

As a result, of these chronic migraine headaches, I had to alter my daily routine by retiring to bed early, on weekdays after work, and I would spend most of my weekends in bed. I can recall how socially disconnected I began to feel. Despite my medical battle with chronic migraines, I remained active in my church and in my career as a Mental Health Qualified Professional.

Saturday, May 5, 2012, was a beautiful spring day, in which I had adequate energy and decided to go to the movies and mall. By the end of the day, I didn't feel good but I wasn't sick enough to visit the emergency room or urgent care. That night I said my prayers and went to bed, as usual. The next morning, I awoke, feeling somewhat dizzy and sweaty, upon standing. I reached for my phone, to inform my sister and some friends, that I wasn't feeling well and I was going to the emergency room. I attempted to get out of my bed but continued to feel dizzy upon standing. I decided to rest in bed, a little longer. A few minutes lapsed and I began to fall asleep. I was eloped by a very peaceful feeling and an odd sensation, that felt as if I had wings and were flying. I then attempted to close my eyes but the phone rang. My sister informed me that she was coming to transport me, to the emergency room. My daughter then entered my bedroom, to assist me, with gathering my belongings, to take to the hospital. I began to experience breathing difficulties or what medical professionals refer to as, Cheyne stokes.

As I had an experience with working with hospice patients and the elderly, so I was familiar with the noises that I was making and became alarmed. I went flailing to my front door but I collapsed in the thresh hole of the door. I continued to have difficulty breathing but I also began to convulse. Although, I was convulsing, I could see that my sister had arrived, at my house and my daughter and son were watching me, as I convulse on the floor. It felt as if everything was moving in slow motion. I could hear my daughter informing 911, of our address. I tried to speak but couldn't. I began to pray in my mind and then suddenly, my prayer language sprang fourth, from out of my mouth and I began to pray in tongues. The EMS arrived and asked, "Can you walk mam?" I responded, "No." The EMS then wrapped me in a sheet and placed me on a stretcher. When I arrived at the hospital, I informed the team of medical professionals, that I hadn't been feeling well and that my symptoms were Cheyne stokes, dizziness, fainting at home, as well as heavy perspiration. I was immediately connected to a heart monitor, IV was started and my blood was drawn. I conversed with the team of medical professionals. Upon the teams exit, I could feel myself slowly going unconscious. I couldn't open my eyes but I could hear the doctor and nurse talking over my head. The doctor said, "They can die at 6." I tried but I still couldn't open my eyes. I then felt the nurse turn me over. I then was able to open my eyes. The nurse stated, "I've got to get you cleaned up." I said, "Why, I'm not dirty?" The nurse explained to me that I had an "accident" and needed to be cleaned up. Meanwhile, I had a visitor. The doctor re-entered the room and reviewed my lab results. The doctor stated, "This can't be right, take it again." Immediately, blood was drawn again, for testing and the results were alarming. The doctor said, "You're being admitted, you're very sick." "Your iron level is a 4 and these numbers are very low." "You have lost a lot of blood and we're going to have to give you a blood transfusion." "You will need about 6 units of blood." I was presented with consent forms, by the hospital representative, to be admitted into the hospital. I provided my signature on the consent forms and was admitted, into the hospital.

After I was admitted, I was taken to the Surgical Triage Intensive Care Unit. I was listed as, "critical condition." Upon my entering the unit, the hospital Chaplain, entered my room. Much to the Chaplains surprise, I was awake and oriented. She presented me with a bible and inquired about my prayer life. I informed her, that I was a Christian and that I have an active prayer life. Upon my improvement in the Surgical Triage Intensive Care Unit, I was transported to a floor in the main hospital, where I spent 4 days. During my stay, I had an endoscopy, which revealed that I had a very tiny ulcer in my stomach, which had bled, when I had taken medication for a migraine headache, on during the previous week. I was unaware, that I had an ulcer, in my stomach. The doctor was surprised, by how tiny the ulcer was and couldn't believe that it caused me to bleed profusely. Upon my discharge from the hospital, my sister stated, "God spoke to me and told me to pick you up and take you to the hospital." The one thing that I know, is that God is always on time and Sunday May 6, 2012 God was more than on time, he was ever present in my time of trouble. No matter how critical the circumstances are, there is always hope, in every situation.

Due to allergic reactions and negative side effects, I'm limited to the medications that I can orally ingest. It became more difficult to remain employed and complete my master's program. At this point, that I was diagnosed with uterine fibroids and again suffered from chronic anemia. I received iron infusions on a regular basis. I was incredibly fatigued but I had a desire to succeed. Foremost, with prayer and God's unfailing love, I completed my master's program and had a hysterectomy in the summer of 2016. I graduated with what most colleges refer to as a, Cum Laude grade point average.

Fibromyalgia is a bio psychosocial disorder, that is either inherited, caused by childhood trauma or accident related. Inevitably, you will never understand my pain, unless you too suffer from fibromyalgia. However, fibromyalgia is more than just aches and pains. The symptoms of fibromyalgia vary from person to person. Some symptoms are: Chronic fatigue, muscular aches, spasms and pains in different areas of the body, tender points, pain that lasts longer than 3 months, joint stiffness, headaches, irritable bowel syndrome, TMJ, nausea, sensitivities, painful menstrual cycles (dysmenorrhea) and brain fog. Individuals with Fibromyalgia experience "flares," in which the pain and symptoms are exacerbated. Flares are caused by weather, hormonal changes, stress, fatigue, accidents or dietary changes.

People with this syndrome experience feelings of loneliness, due to the chronic fatigue and pain, which cause them to isolate themselves, from their friends and families. People with this debilitating syndrome need the proper bed rest.

I have learned how to manage the symptoms of fibromyalgia by utilizing prayer, eating dietary supplements such as turmeric, getting the proper rest, minimizing stress levels on the job and in my personal life. I know that I am on a journey to healing. I no longer suffer from chronic anemia and I am free from fibroids.

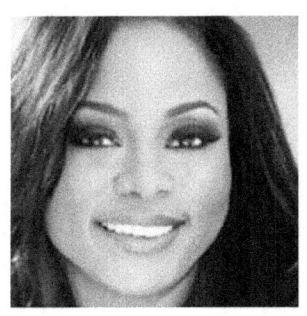

Antonia Perkins-bio

Antonia Perkins was born in Macon, Georgia on August 19, 1973. She received her Bachelors of Arts degree with a major in Criminal Justice and a minor in Theatre Arts, from The University of North Carolina at Wilmington in 2005 and the Master of Arts degree in Mental Health Counseling in 2016, from Webster University. Antonia began her career, in the mental health field in 2006 and has held various positions various positions. She is also a professional actress and is represented by Maultsby Talent, in which she was a top ten nominee in Hollywood's Best New Talent competition in 2008.

Chapter Six

THIS BABY WILL LIVE AND NOT DIE

Lakeisha Martin

I married my pastor husband on January 22, 2000. And I have since learned that we must be careful of the words that we speak into the atmosphere. The Bible tells us "What you say can mean life or death. Those who speak with care will be rewarded." Proverbs 18:21 (New Century Version). I had always been one to say "When I get married, I don't want any children for at least five to seven years. I just want to enjoy my husband." I didn't know those words would put me in one of the hardest fights of my life: a 13-year long battle with infertility. We tried for years to have a child, but nothing would happen. My gynecologist couldn't figure it out. He said I should be getting pregnant; your weight may be an issue, but you should be getting pregnant. Month after month, nothing would happen. After years of being unsuccessful with my him, we began going to fertility doctors.

My first miscarriage happened in 2005 at just five weeks. We went to the doctor to have our first ultrasound and was told there was no heartbeat.

Just a few short months later, we conceived using fertility medicine and got pregnant with triplets. We were overjoyed! When we heard those three tiny heartbeats on the monitor, my husband stomped his foot, threw back his head, and laughed. We couldn't believe how fortunate we were. We didn't know how we would care for three children, but we weren't worried about it!

I lost those children at 23.5 weeks. My husband had to work late so I was home alone. I was laying in the bed watching television and felt like I had to use the bathroom. I got up and a little water ran down my leg. It wasn't a huge amount, so I wasn't worried. But then a little more water. By that time, my husband had made it home and I told him what was happening. After water coming down my leg for the third time, we decided to call the doctor. The nurse assured us that we were probably all right but with three babies inside, one of them was bound to kick my bladder sooner or later. But after dropping what I now know was my mucus plug, we headed to the hospital.

For no apparent reason, I went into spontaneous labor and delivered my first daughter stillborn. Her face and body were dark and bruised due to the contractions on her way out, but we could tell she looked just like her mommy. I delivered her on January 21, 2006. One day before my sixth wedding anniversary.

I had two babies left inside so we were ready to fight for their lives. Our doctors decided to try something called the Trendelenburg position. This was where they took my bed and almost stood me on my head to try and make the other babies stay in my womb. I was also still contracting so our doctors decided to give me a combination of medicines to try and stop the contractions. I can't remember all of what I had but one I'll never forget was magnesium. I'll explain why in a moment.

As all of this is taking place in the hospital, my husband and I were mainly alone except for two to three close family members and a close family friend. We are private people, so we never really shared with anyone the true struggle we were having. All anyone knew was that I was pregnant. The friend I mentioned is a dear sweet sister, who is also a psalmist, and had been believing with me for children. She came and stayed with me one night and she and I began to do what we always did: worship God. We closed our eyes and sang until the Holy Ghost began to sing through us. We sang for almost an hour and we absolutely forgot where we were. As the peace of God settled right there among us, we didn't know the effect it was having on my tiny section of that big hospital. When we opened our eyes, my room was filled with nurses, doctors, and other patients who were crying with uplifted hands. They were weeping, worshipping, and crying out to God for their own situations. And as I look back on that time, I understand God even more now. I didn't know it then, but the worship brought us strength for what we were about to face.

Nobody told us that we were going to lose those babies. And I believe our doctors did the best they could, but I also believe they knew the truth. One night while trying to sleep, laying almost on my head, I began to experience something. Remember I said I'll never forget that one of the drugs I was taking was magnesium? Well here's why. I couldn't figure out if I was awake, asleep, or somewhere in between but I saw my husband's face smiling at me. It kept getting smaller and smaller and it was like I was falling into a dark hole. I tried to call out to him as he lay asleep next to me but I had no voice. I felt as if I was leaving the earth. I silently asked God to help me to do something and He allowed me to eke out my husband's name ever so softly, "Anthony." It was a whisper, but he awoke immediately out of his sleep. I motioned for him to get somebody and when the doctors came in, they began to move frantically because I was only breathing 32% on my own. The magnesium they had given me to stop the contractions had begun to fill up in my lungs and I couldn't breathe!

They had to get me stabilized with methods including an oxygen tent. And because I couldn't breathe, neither could my babies. So, I had to deliver another daughter and son who looked just like my husband. They came out perfectly formed just too tiny to live. They were laboring to breathe and although they were crying, no sound came out because their voices hadn't yet developed. See the thing about multiples, they develop a lot slower than a single child, and it is against the law to give a baby less than 24 week of normal gestational age, a steroid to help their lungs develop. As the doctors were saving my life, my beautiful children were dying. They only lived for about three hours before dying in my husband's arms. I never got to spend any time with them. This was on January 24, 2006. Two days after my sixth wedding anniversary.

We will never forget our sweet nurses. They knew it was our anniversary and made us a card that they all signed. They wrote personal notes inside the card saying things like they've never seen stronger people or that they've never experienced God's love like they had while tending to us. They told us they actually "fought" among each other to see who would work extra shifts just to care for us! I truly believe in angels on earth and believe some were summoned to us in that hospital. But even though we were suffering loss, we were still representing and sharing Jesus!

Throughout all of this, we told no one about our infertility issues. People knew we weren't pregnant anymore, but they didn't know the depths of our struggle, about what really happened to me in that hospital bed, or how my husband NEVER once closed the church doors or missed a service. He didn't talk to anybody about his heart. He kept moving by faith and God's strength which is something I still admire about him to this day. That was how he made it through. But for me it was different. I wasn't where he was. See after I healed physically, I went right back to teaching and preaching but I never shared my heart with anyone and I needed to talk! I needed to open up but I really didn't know how or to whom. I didn't have a best friend or a sisterhood that I could lean on. Even my friend from the hospital didn't know everything. I only had my husband and he was struggling too. We comforted each other as best we could and although it wasn't easy, I believe that is why our marriage is so strong today.

I remember being on autopilot that whole year. I still can't remember things because I was so numb. I never thought I would walk into that hospital pregnant and happy and barely walk out alive and with no children. Of course, it caused me to struggle in my faith! But as a leader, and a strong one, people look up to you for strength and encouragement. But how do the leaders get the same thing for themselves? I preached some powerful messages during that time on faith and expectation. And it blessed the people tremendously. I saw God move on their behalves. But in all honesty, those messages didn't help me much. I was in survival mode. I knew what to do so I did it. End of story. I had to keep going. But do you want to know what truly kept me humble and my heart soft towards God? My prayer life. I needed someone in this earthly realm but I'm so glad I didn't close my heart to my Heavenly Father! I was brutally honest with Him. I told Him how hurt I was and how I didn't understand. Some days I was comforted and some days I was not.

I got pregnant again in 2007 this time with twin boys. The doctors diagnosed me with a weakened cervix and said this was probably my issue all along. As you can tell, I had no problem getting pregnant I just couldn't stay pregnant! So, they said I needed something called a cerclage which is a stitch at the base of the cervix to keep it closed. It was supposed to help hold the weight of the pregnancy and to allow me to carry to term. I had the cerclage put in place at three months pregnant and was in labor by four months pregnant. The culprit this time? An infection. I didn't receive any antibiotics after my procedure and went into spontaneous labor again.

Because of the stitch, the boys broke through my cervix causing major blood loss. I labored all day in pain, bleeding excessively, knowing that I was again going to lose my children. It finally happened, and I gave birth to two stillborn boys. This time, I told my husband to go home, get some rest, and I would be fine. We'd been here before, I'm strong, and I'll be okay. There I went again with that "Superwoman" mentality! He didn't want to go but reluctantly agreed and left promising to be back soon.

As soon as he left, I found out that because of the blood loss, I needed multiple transfusions. But for reasons I can't remember I was so scared to receive the blood. Doctors and nurses kept coming in asking me to sign the papers, so we could get everything started, telling me I was wasting time, and that I needed to decide. They said my organs were beginning to shut down because of the lack of blood but I still wouldn't sign for the transfusions. I don't know what was going through my mind because if this happened to me today, I wouldn't even think twice about signing those papers.

One strong-willed nurse kept coming in asking me when my husband would be back. I kept telling her he'd be back soon. Boy she was persistent. A few hours later she came in with a different set of papers stating that by my signature, I knew I was declining the blood, and could possibly die. She locked eyes with me and said, "Before you sign, call your husband." I agreed, and she stood there as I told my husband the situation. And if I got something wrong, she quickly corrected me and just would not leave my bedside. I now thank God for her! Hearing my husband's voice snapped me back into reality. He sweetly but firmly told me to sign because he couldn't go through losing more children and this time his wife as well. My God!

As they hooked me up for the transfusions, I lay there asking God if I had done something wrong, and was I worthy to be a mother. You can imagine how my heart was breaking into pieces. But He never did answer.

I got pregnant a few more times and lost them all. We believe that if we had all the children that were conceived, we would have about nine kids in total! My last pregnancy was ectopic (implanted in my tube and couldn't possibly survive) and would not absolve itself. My doctor kept waiting and hoping it would, but we had a time limit of how long we could wait before the tube would burst. We even tried a cancer drug called methotrexate to attack the cells and bring the pregnancy to an end. Unfortunately, the medicine didn't work either, but it did a number on my body. It was almost as if I were a cancer patient myself. I lost my hair, developed dark circles around my eyes, and even got open wounds on my inner thighs that I could put my fingers down into. My tube did eventually burst which is what ultimately brought that pregnancy to an end.

Throughout all of this, we kept preaching and teaching. We kept the doors of our church open and continued pushing others to greatness. After all, this is the call on our lives and we had to uphold the mandate. But no one really knew the pain I endured or the heaviness of the shame and grief I carried. Although one day while I was in prayer, I repented to God. It's just like a switch went off in my head and I told Him how sorry I was for allowing childbearing to take my attention all those previous years. He actually warned me years earlier, but I didn't heed the warning. He spoke to my heart saying anything, no matter how good it is, when used in or desired in excess, could become a plague. I still didn't understand that fully though.

Listen, I could have died twice. I asked my husband for a divorce on two different occasions and thankfully he paid my requests no attention. I was so busy in my pain that I couldn't see how blessed I truly was in so many other ways. I began to share with God in my prayer time that I understood that people didn't always get the things or outcomes that they prayed for and I accepted and was okay with that. Let me tell you, when you stop fighting against the waves and begin to swim with the flow, it's a lot easier. Our church was thriving spiritually and honestly so was I. My relationship with God had become so solid through all of this; He never let me go. I didn't have a hardened heart towards Him and He was taking my life in directions I'd never dreamed imaginable for me. I went back to school, began to lose weight, and my husband and I began to take vacations. Us! We had never left or closed the church doors in almost a decade. We began to fully enjoy our lives.

One particular day, I was washing dishes and praying. It had been a few years since that ectopic and I was in a great place spiritually, mentally, and emotionally. The Lord Himself began speaking to me at that kitchen sink and told me that I would conceive again and this time, I would have the child. The baby would be a boy and I would name him Anthony Jr. but give him the nickname of "AntJay." The significance of this was that I was going to birth a man child with the traits and spirit of his earthly father but that he was also going to be an individual force to be reckoned with for the Lord! After He finished speaking to my heart, I began to worship and praise Him. I had no trace of fear, miscarriage, or doubt because I knew God's voice and I believed Him!

By the time my husband got home, I had moved on to cleaning the refrigerator, and I didn't even hear him come in. I had some praise music on with earbuds in my ear and Anthony said that I was on one leg dancing in that kitchen! He said the atmosphere was so charged with the presence of God that he knew God had spoken a word to me. I shared with him what I'd heard, and we believed.

I need to tell you something right here. It didn't happen overnight. And by this time, I was already in my late thirties. I had lost over 100 pounds and was by far in the best shape spiritually and physically than I'd ever been in my life. But don't you think the enemy didn't TRY to put fear and doubt in my heart. Did God really say that? Will I really have this child? Remember what happened before? I had to pray, fast for endurance, and remember what the Lord had spoken to me in my kitchen. It wasn't always easy, and my heart would sometimes be tempted to give in to the doubt, but I had to hold on to the promise! I had to believe God even when it looked like the promise wasn't going to come. See, there's a space and time between the promise and the pregnancy. And it was there, in that space, that my faith was tried. I didn't know when it would happen. But because of all those days and nights of prayer, no matter how long it took, I knew it would.

I learned a beautiful thing about a consistent prayer life and keeping a journal. I could always pray for strength and go back and read the words I'd pen in my journal. I had been keeping journals since I was 12 years old. But I can always tell now when I'm writing and when Holy Spirit takes over. The sentences, wording, and thoughts are so different when it's Him speaking. How do I know that? Because no matter how spiritual I am, I could never pen it more beautifully, accurately, or clearly as the Holy Spirit can!

Needless to say, because the promise came from the Lord, we are the proud parents of an almost five-year-old son! No fertility medicines, no special tricks, just standing on a promise from our Lord and Savior. I went from a little girl sleeping on the floor at her Grandmother's house to a woman preaching and teaching God's Gospel to those who would and sometimes wouldn't listen. But this wasn't about all that at this point in my life. This was my personal faith walk, journey, testimony-builder. How could I preach and teach to others if I myself didn't wholeheartedly believe? My infertility battle was a long and hard one, believe me. But God is absolutely who He says

He is and because I had gotten to know Him intimately, I knew I could trust Him. I'd hoped, dreamed, believed, and lost but He was still my God. Even when I didn't understand, He was my God. When He would be silent when I prayed for answers, He was still my God. The battle fine-tuned my faith for that level and that's how I could fully receive the promise with no fear.

When we got pregnant, our new OB/GYN asked if we wanted to have all those tests they want to administer when a woman is over 35 years of age. My immediate answer was no. You may wonder how I could be so sure and think shouldn't I have done it just to be sure? I WAS SURE! This promise was spoken to me by Him and nothing was going to hinder it from coming to pass. I bless God for leading me to a new Christian doctor because when I told her no, she grabbed my hands and we prayed right there in her office for a safe and problem free pregnancy and delivery with a healthy child. Case closed!

My son is an absolute joy. I enjoyed carrying him. I enjoyed singing to him in my belly. As a matter of fact, I am the praise and worship leader at my church and I never sat down from service. I was leading praise and worship the Sunday before I went into labor late Monday the next night. Singing was and still is my joy. It keeps me close to the Lord. I love when I can sing to Him and He be an audience of One. I love to worship and laugh and that's what I did throughout my entire pregnancy. I think that's why AntJay loves to sing with me now and why he keeps his mommy laughing. He's hilarious!

My pregnancy was easy too. I only gained 14 pounds initially but shot up to 19 pounds two weeks before delivery. I didn't want the birth to be videoed, but my husband snuck his phone in and captured it anyway. I'm so glad he did! I was only in labor for six minutes and after three focused pushes, my promise was here! You can hear the nurse ask, "Who giggles while giving birth?" I didn't even have to answer. My doctor spoke up saying something to the effect of if you only knew what they'd been through you would know why God has this room filled with joy overflowing!

My sister, please don't give up on God. He has a specific plan for your life. And although you may not know what it is, He does. According to Jeremiah 29:11, it's already arranged. But don't just stop at that verse. Please take it from me. Prayer is vital and much needed to overcome the tests, trials, and tribulations of this life. If you don't keep connected with your Heavenly Father, you absolutely will not make it! If you have a prayer life and a hunger for His Word, you will win!

Let me leave you with a few verses of scripture and my utmost blessing upon your life. Whatever you may be going through, know that God has a plan and a purpose for you. Sis, dig into prayer, push your plate back and fast, journal if you're so inclined. But whatever you do, don't run FROM the Lord, run TO Him! Keep your heart softened so you may hear Him when He speaks.

[11] I say this because I know what I am planning for you," says the Lord. "I have good plans for you, not plans to hurt you. I will give you hope and a good future. [12] Then you will call my name. You will come to me and pray to me, and I will listen to you. [13] You will search for me. And when you search for me with all your heart, you will find me! [14] I will let you find me," says the Lord..." – Jeremiah 29:11-14 (New Century Version)

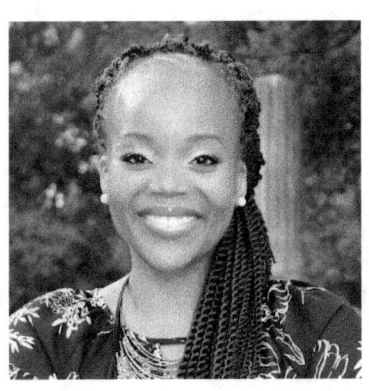

Lakeisha Martin-Bio

Lady Lakeisha Martin was born in Nyack, New York and was raised by her dearly departed Grandmother. At just 19 years of age, she moved to Tuscaloosa, Alabama in June 1996. She was introduced to a church by a co-worker and it was there that she met Minister Anthony L. Martin. Unbeknownst to her, she would later marry him in January 2000, and together just eight short months later, they would become the founders of Victory Pentecostal Holiness Church in Tuscaloosa, Alabama.

Lady Martin is known as a woman of prayer, psalmist, loving wife, doting mother, and loyal friend. She's been preaching since the age of 27 and some of her most memorable messages tackle what we all struggle with today: marriage and family, faith, and maintaining a consistent prayer life. She knows that God has anointed her to speak life into His women to restore their confidence, to empower them to stand, and to accept their gifts and callings in life whatever they may be.

Lady and Pastor Martin have been married for almost 19 beautiful years and counting. And from this union, they have "faithed-in" one handsome, four-year-old baby boy, named

Anthony L. Martin, Jr., whom they affectionately call "AntJay." One of the reasons why Lady Martin's ministry, prayer life, and walk with God is so strong and anointed is because she and her husband endured a 13-year long struggle with infertility. Through this trying of her faith, she knows beyond a shadow of a doubt that God is real, and this allows her to speak with passion, power, and invoke a call to action in others. AntJay is one of the greatest joys in their lives!

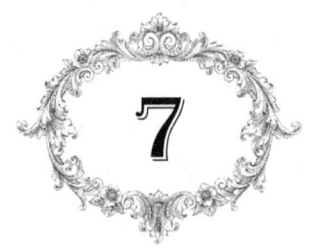

Chapter Seven

ANOINTED AND DEPRESSED

Ikisha Cross

My name is Ikisha S. Cross and this is my story...

Born in Cheverly, Maryland, and raised in Washington, D.C., I lived in the inner city where crime, poverty and hopelessness was the norm. My strong mother raised my siblings and me, refusing to succumb to her surroundings and fighting to create a better life for us. She succeeded, but it came with a cost.

I grew up in church. I was saved and baptized at the tender age of nine years old. I did it because I believed it was the right thing to do, and my grandma said so. I served on the Youth Usher Board and sang in the children's choir. I later joined my mother's church. Knowing everything about church that there was to know, I somehow always felt like something was missing. I never felt like I fit or belonged. I fought tirelessly to fit in and to be a part but just couldn't do it.

Aside from fitting in, I was also trying to understand, for many years, why multiple men, who I was supposed to trust, sexually violated me. I also questioned why my "unknown" father wasn't in my life and learned later that it was to protect me. I often asked myself "What was wrong with me?" These events and contemplations pushed me into a dark place that I gradually believed was normal.

After the abuse stopped, I built walls to protect myself. The thought of allowing someone to get too close bothered me. I did not want anyone to know my shame or to see my reality because I define myself by my abuse and scars. I was damaged goods — violated and unclaimed by the men who were supposed to make me feel safe. My attitudes toward relationships with men were poisoned and jaded. I had no real understanding of how to maintain a loving, caring relationship with a man once I didn't and couldn't trust them.

Unhealed, I married in 2005 while seven months pregnant with my son. I walked down the aisle, feeling as big as a house. I was ashamed and embarrassed — a spectacle. With many doubts, I married because I wanted to give my baby what I didn't have — a two-parent family. With all the joy that came from his birth, I still found myself in that very dark place.

It was almost as if a dark cloud hovered over me, and I would cry for hours on end, not wanting to move or get up and care for my baby. I know that sounds like postpartum depression, and it was. But beyond counseling and the support of family, this darkness seemed very familiar to me, like an old lover, who knew me and I knew him. So I'd go to church, get prayer, fall out, shout, dance and believe that God would take away the bad feelings. I expected them to fall off, so I wouldn't have to deal with them. I was hoping they would magically disappear.

For a while, I was great, feeling happy and free; only to realize, I was still bound. The darkness didn't fall off or disappear!!! It was waiting for me to put it on like a robe and slippers after every shout, dance and falling out. I didn't want to acknowledge this darkness; I only wanted to believe it didn't exist. Unfortunately, I soon returned to it because it was all I knew.

Fast-forward to 2007 when I experienced a very public church divorce. I felt sad and lonely but still managed to get out of bed for all three church services each Sunday. I was still singing in the choir, serving, and attending church meetings because that's what I was told to do. It helped me function; it kept me busy; but it didn't allow me to address my new reality. I was moving and pushing, but not healing. I avoided dealing with the added tragedy and grief that came with divorce because I had to ignore it. In my mind, confronting it was weak. The potential emotions and tears showed weakness. If I buckled under all of this pressure, then I WAS WEAK.

At this time, my relationship with God was very surface. I knew God's power; I had seen it; but I didn't know it would work for or through me. The way I allowed people to mistreat me was how I defined God's feelings toward me. I questioned, "Why would His power work for me or through me? I wasn't worthy." I relied heavily on those around me to tell me what to do. They were the voice of God in my life, not God himself. So when they said to gird myself up and stop crying over the mess I made, or to get myself together because I only wanted attention, or that I was being overly dramatic, I suppressed my gloom and dread, pretending they were nonexistent. When they told me to "pull on the power in me", I wondered, "What power?" I was certain that God would never speak to me because I wasn't important enough, I came from the wrong part of town and I had done the unthinkable. Please don't assume that my advisors were bad people because they're not; they were simply giving me what they knew to be sound wisdom.

By August 2013, I was experiencing a part of life that I had only heard about beforehand: they called it "rock bottom". I had lost loved ones, my marriage, my home and my lucrative job. I was employed for less than what I was accustomed to and could barely keep a roof over my and my son's heads. Transition after transition, I had never experienced this kind of pain or sadness, and it all happened at once without any breaks. This rock bottom was like a new, fresh hell.

For many years, I hid behind serving in and/or leading several ministries in my local church; but after each service, meeting or church event, I would go home alone and fight unexplainable sadness, insecurity, self-doubt, self-hatred, frustration and anger. I repeatedly questioned whether I would ever be good enough, pretty enough and strong enough, and whether I could ever live up to their expectations.

Would I ever become what I've seen or will I always continue to be good enough to serve and not be minimized by those I serve? Their treatment convinced me that I would never be good enough to accomplish the things that I knew God had called me to and had for me. I eventually realized that I wasn't just emotional; I was depressed, church going, shouting, speaking in tongues, anointed, called, chosen AND DEPRESSED!! SICK WITH DEPRESSION!!! Thoughts of my future gave me anxiety. I thought many times, THIS IS IT!!! The kind of depression that made me wonder "why am I still here?" "why stay here"? "why would God want me"? I was broken! Wearing the "mask", quoting the church clichés but I was dying inside.

I would go home and cry for hours and even contemplate suicide; made a few attempts because I felt like no one including God loved me or really understood what I was experiencing. I felt ashamed to go to anyone because here I am a leader in the church but can't control my emotions. I was told that I needed to navigate my emotions, and get them in check, nothing I was dealing with was that bad, I was unstable and double minded and could potentially affect people. I lived a life of fear, torment and panic.

I learned to live with it and hide it to avoid feeling judged, minimized and embarrassed. I learned to be someone else. I developed the ability to show people who I wanted them to see resulting in me having NO idea of who I was. I had become a deceiver; solely to hide my brokeness . I was unable to show emotions unless it was anger. I was hard, resentful, unforgiving, doubtful, coarse, unapproachable, untrusting and callus. I did not trust the soul of anyone; everyone had a motive; men. Most of them I used because they numbed me.. I questioned everything and would always lean to the negative FIRST. I was pessimistic, envious and jealous of people. Jealous of their freedom because I desired to be free, but I was STUCK!!!

I was ashamed of who I was privately but prideful publically. I hated myself!!! I hated life!!! I hated the "church" because no one saw how broken I was or they just didn't care. To them I was a commodity of servanthood and I needed to get myself together. I got tired of hearing how anointed I was and how God had a plan for my life. It sickened me!!! I could care less about how anointed I was and how He'd use me, I was trying to make it to the next minute without having a breakdown. I didn't care about the anointing, I wanted to know how the heck do I navigate through life!!! I wanted to know how to get FREE!

My defining moment was in 2013 when I obeyed the voice of God and transitioned to another ministry. Not because my previous church was bad but because it was time to go, to heal , to grow, to meet myself and that's exactly what happened. The process began in August 2013 when I lost my home and was evicted. I stood in the middle of the courtyard looking at all of the things I had work so hard for laying in the grass. It broke me, but I made myself pull it together. I slept on my best friend's couch with my child for 5 months. During that time, I lost a dear friend and relative, due to the SAME lie and stress that had taken over my life.The lie of everything being ok and I really am happy. I worked 12-15 hour days just to avoid everything. . I was not sleeping; I was not eating. I was functioning like a robot. . This pattern continued until October of 2013. I was walking down the hallway with my brother and they tell me I was talking randomly, nothing I said was making any sense. They took my son into the house and my brother looked at me and said let it fall apart.

Break!!! I was told I said "I'm fine" and that I had to get in the house to take care of my child. I eventually collapsed and started screaming and crying. I heard my brother in my ear telling me to cry and "let it all out!" and he held me up let me cry in his arms. I was tired, I was weak, I was exhausted, I WAS SICK!!! I learned how to live with to happen to move me to freedom. Sick of keeping up appearances, sick of pretending to be ok, sick of with lying, sick of hurting, sick of hiding, I was sick!!! I realized I had no thoughts of the future because I had no idea who I was. I had no idea I, Ikisha, had a future that God Himself created for me, not the me that everyone wanted me to be, but the me He designed! A free me!! A healed me!! A delivered me!! I was sick and the sickness of depression and loss of self-identity caused me to become someone I was not.

I was lying because I was SICK, I was promiscuous because I was SICK, I was overeating because I was SICK, I overworked because I was SICK. I did anything I could think of to not have to deal with that deep darkness that was inside of me. Anything to numb it, anything that would make it go away even for a little while. I medicated myself not with drugs but with men, with church, with my career. I just wanted it to stop; I wanted clarity of thought; I wanted peace of mind; I wanted to SLEEP!

Yes, I knew God called me but I didn't care, because my "call" wasn't keeping me. I needed the thing that keeps you. I had come into a place of desiring freedom more than anything. I was desperate! I just wanted to be free! My Pastor saw it. He saw the mask; He saw my prison. He did not take advantage of my issues; instead he allowed me to come to church, sit, hear God's Word and ushered me into the process of gaining my freedom. He forced me to sit and heal. I cried; I screamed; I yelled; I prayed. My Pastor gave me the space to get what I needed and not be concerned with leading. Most importantly he didn't lead me to him; he sent me back to God. By this time I had become a slave to unforgiveness, bitterness, anger, fear, anxiety, and pride. I had learned to live with this stuff; it kept me bound and unable to move in the purpose of God. I was chained to this stuff.

I FINALLY surrendered one night at home. I was tired, and worn out. So I began to worship; I told Him how much I loved him and how I needed him; I told Him how tired I was and how I just wanted to be free. I told God what I wanted to hear someone say about me. Then I heard these words, "I have always wanted you", "I have always loved you." Imagine me encountering a loving Father who wanted to be where I was and to ensure me that He loved and wanted me. The presence of God came and found me and held me in the dark place of my mind and comforted me. That was the first time I remember feeling safe. I previously rejected a serious relationship with God because of fear. I had been mishandled by men so many times. In my mind God was a man and He would drop me just like they did; but I was wrong. He taught me FIRST that He would never drop me. Through prayer and study He taught me how to face those demons that had tormented me for years; He made me acknowledge them and held my hand through it. He gave me space to talk about how badly it hurt me. I would go to the Father and cry, sometimes screaming; only having the words "it hurts", "they hurt me", "where were You" not knowing that those cries and screams were healing me. The Lord taught me that tears are not a sign of weakness but a sign of strength and that He had been storing every last tear and saving them just He said He would in Psalm 56.

He was healing me. I realized that although He knew anyway, He just wanted me to trust Him enough to tell Him; He wanted the pain and shame but it was hard because I had held on to for so many years and just didn't know how to let it go. He gave me the courage to give it to Him. When I realized He loved me and would never throw me away; I found myself giving Him everything. Things I pushed so deep inside of me that I forgot they were there. This exchange birthed intercession in my life. I had learned to call on God. Previously taught by my spiritual mother but never put into practice. After a year my Pastor felt the release from God and loosed me to pray and intercede in the house. In 2015 I was licensed to preach the gospel and affirmed as a prophet in the Lord's church; ONLY after I sat and allowed God to heal me. My Pastor allowed me to SIT! Not lead, not serve, he let me heal. I will forever be grateful to him for that.

In February 2016 after ending an unhealthy relationship, I met someone who would change my life. They were interested in learning who I was and not who once pretended to be. I was able to share my faults and what was once my shame and they showed God's heart for me. They loved me, encouraged me, they protected me, loved my son and cared for him in a way I had not seen anyone do outside of my family. They vowed to do this for the rest of our lives.

On September 10th I married the man of dreams. When this book is published we would have just celebrated our 2-year anniversary and in July of 2018 welcomed our beautiful little girl. I have a family with a man that loves me JUST LIKE I AM!

Today I am Free!! I am walking in freedom, I live in freedom!! I am walking out my healing. I live in my healing. I breathe in my healing. I am healed in my mind. I am healed in my soul. I am healed in my spirit. I am healed in my emotions. God has healed me. God is healing me. I have no fear of the future because my future is in God's hands and because I know Him and

He loves me there are promises over my life. So I can walk into the future with NO FEAR! I understand and know that I am loved, I am worthy, and I am important to God and SO ARE YOU!

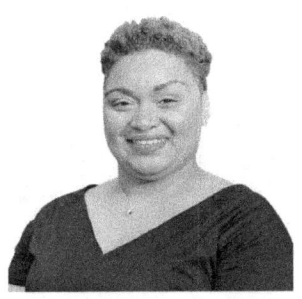

Prophet Ikisha S. Cross-Bio

Ikisha Cross Is an ordained minister and a prophetic voice in Cleburne, Texas Her life is a perfect example of the "Overcomer." She is not ashamed to tell her REAL story, Ikisha lives by Revelations 12:11 "And they overcame him by the blood of the Lamb, and by the word of their testimony" and by Hebrews 11:1 Now Faith is the substances of things hope for, the evidence of things not seen." She is conduit of change. Ikisha encourages all she comes in contact with to be fearless in their pursuit of the things of God. Ikisha has more than a decade of teaching and counseling, which enables her to reach others with Transparency, Honesty, Humor, Warmth and strength. She is married to the love of her of life Prophet Kirklin Cross Jr. and the mother of 4 beautiful children; Judah, Aniyah, Daelyn and Kellan. She is a wife, mother, author, teacher and a mentor but above all is she is SAVED!!!

Chapter Eight

ESCAPING TOXICITY

Suprena Hickman

A hospital is a place where you can go for healing, however, you can become more ill as a result of your exposure and stay. In the hospital or medical facility, this is called a nosocomial infection. Some call them "super bugs" because they are difficult to treat due to the bodies building up resistance to them, then the body becomes very toxic. Just imagine being ill, and going to a place where you know healing occurs, then becoming more ill. Now, imagine having to be there daily, providing care for others who are ill, and you become increasingly toxic due to your surroundings. Well, allow me to share what happened to me.

I was enjoying my life as a young travel nurse. I was blessed to be able to work for travel agencies and visit different cities and states while doing what I did best at that time. I was attracted to the travel nursing niche because of the freedom it provided. It was also quite lucrative for a floor nurse. As a traveler, we were mission focused. We came in, took care of our patients and helped out the unit, then kept it moving. If we made friends along the way, then thats great. We didn't get caught up in the politics of the facility. We were just the help. So, why did I stop traveling if I loved it so much is what you may be wondering, huh? It's a question I often asked myself during this time.

Well, I was heavily influenced at that time by friends, coworkers, and family members who kept telling me that I needed to get a real job. Despite the fact that I had a great paying job, with benefits, and amazing flexibility, I listened to them telling me to get a real job. So, I decided to do the "adult thing" and get a "real job" as I was being told. I applied and interviewed for a clinical nurse position in a government medical facility and was immediately hired. I finally had the nine-to-five job with federal benefits and I didn't have to work weekends anymore. After spending twelve years working nearly every weekend, this was a relief. I remember being excited about starting something new, but I was definitely thinking about the travel assignment to Hawaii that I was planning to take with another fellow Nurse. Everyone around me seemed excited for me and celebrated my success, however, deep down inside, I really wasn't happy. I even took a pay cut to get this job. So many feelings and thoughts were going through my head. I also had deep regrets for not standing up for myself and telling my loved ones that I loved what I was doing.

Well, from the time I was hired for this new job, there were many problems for me. It seemed as if everything that could go wrong actually did. The hiring process actually took a few months from the time I accepted the position to the first day starting the job. The communication during that time was very poor. I wasn't able to accept another travel assignment because I didn't know when I would be starting the new job. No matter how often I called to ask, I was never given a start date. I was able to get some temporary work with my agency while I waited, but I wasn't able to take another contracted assignment. My income decreased tremendously, and my debts seemed to get greater. I was also in school finishing my masters degree at that time and my husband and I were only a couple of years in our new house. I was the "bread winner" in the home and what I was feeling was a bit new. However, I continued the path because I figured it was just the process as I was told many times while calling to inquire if I had really been hired. Yes, it was that bad.

    Nevertheless, months passed by and I finally received a start date. I started with orientation the first week. By the end of that week, I was seriously asking myself what I had gotten into. It was so disorganized, and definitely not challenging of my skillsets- as I was a highly skilled nurse who was critical care trained. I was accustomed to quick movements, quick adaptations to my surroundings due to frequent environmental changes, and quick orientations! I recall us spending two to three days on simply learning how to log in the computerized system and making sure everyone had access. How wasteful and completely boring! You see, as a traveler, there is no time to spend weeks on orientations. My job was to come in, quickly adapt, take care of the patients assigned to me, and keep it moving. I definitely didn't like this new job already, but I was grateful for the opportunity. Therefore, I tried to adjust to the dysfunctions and stick it out. I found myself quickly in trouble within the first three weeks of working this job the I've waited for months to start. Who does that? I've experienced anywhere from hazing and bullying, to having my privacy violated, to inappropriate nurse managers, and I've even being accused of stealing government time! I then realized that I was working amongst a bunch of grown kids in a professional setting. This was different from what I've ever experienced.

You are probably guessing that I didn't stay there long right? WRONG! I truly believed that I needed to suck it up and make it work. So, I put on a smile and made myself celebrate and tolerate this toxic environment for five whole years! Absolutely insane! During those years, I was irritated, angry, and started becoming more bitter and resentful, each day. I nearly walked away from my marriage, my home, and I even became severely ill. During my five years there, I began experiencing prolonged menstrual cycles that would last anywhere from two weeks at a time and began progressing to months with severe abdominal cramping. I was so toxic! So, how would one treat this "super bug"?

I recall going to the doctor for help and my female gynecologist, at that time, was only focused on my obesity. The more I spoke about my discomfort and issues, the more she kept telling me I needed to lose weight and that would take care of most of the problems I had. It seemed as if every direction I turned to for help where I lived, I just couldn't get someone to actually pay attention to my cry out for help and provide me with options. Here I was a registered nurse, walking in the medical facilities for help and now walking out with more pills. They diagnosed me with uterine fibroids and then said, it's common in African-American women. Because I was so toxic, things I would normally think of, I found that I couldn't think. It got to a point where I was literally hemorrhaging and passing

HUGE blood clots as if I was having a miscarriage, but my doctors only seemed to see an obese woman before them when I came for help. At one visit, my primary care doctor saw that I gained more weight since my last visit and she quickly mentioned, before she walked out of the door, that I needed to "just stop eating". I was beyond hurt, became more angry, felt helpless, yet I still was determined to keep moving forward because that's all I knew to do. The medications I was on caused hormonal imbalances and fluid retention, so my weight kept increasing. These were miserable times for me, no doubt. There were many times when I had to cough or sneeze, and the pressure from that, literally caused what was like an explosion from Hell in my uterus. It was an instant blood bath with a series of expelling large clots that looked like raw pieces of liver accompanied with extreme uterine cramping. Oh, and if I had a tampon inserted with the doubled pads I wore, then the tampon would come out with the clot expulsions.

If you are frowned up as you are reading this, then just imagine it happening to you. Just imagine how I felt living like this for a couple of years and still called to coach and counsel other women, have wellness retreats for women, and put on fundraising events for hundreds in the community. Imagine the preparation that was required daily for me to simply leave the house. I traveled with backup clothing, boxes of tampons, pads, bags, and cleaning supplies. I was pumped up on steroids and hormonal drugs, along with a bag of medications- including prescription iron, prescription vitamin D, thyroid medications, water pills, injections, and so much more. I LIVED in the bathrooms wherever I went. As soon as I walked in any building, I needed to know where the bathrooms were located. In addition to my daily hemorrhaging, I had chronic swelling of my limbs, excessive sluggishness, very little energy due to having little to no iron in my body, and I was battling depression. I also had asthma since I was a child, and during these times, with me battling anemia due to the fibroids, I experienced extreme shortness of breath and wheezing. It was difficult to determine if it was asthma related or not. A simple walk from my front door to my car would be exhausting. I would have bursted in perspirations and would have to stop walking for a few minutes to catch my breath. I felt as if I was pulling a car with me every time I walked- and I felt like this while taking prescription iron pills! The toxicity was draining me. You see, fibroids can grow individually or in clusters, so you can have multiple fibroids- as I did. I had one "massive" tumor greater than fifteen centimeters and another large tumor. Amongst these two were "numerous lesions" throughout my uterus. Talk about toxicity!

I've tried various traditional and nontraditional medicine options. Some helped and some didn't. By the time I started the natural products for healing, it helped a little, but it was a bit too late. I remember getting so weak that I got out of bed and went straight to the floor. I remember crying helplessly for God to help me. I wondered how was it that I was able to help heal the sick as a nurse, and also coach women needing healing and direction, but unable to heal myself. Many days, I felt as if I would just die. I was in a doctor's office every week, for something. I was taking a bag of medications daily. I was still working out as much as I could until I felt tightness in my chest as I inhaled with every movement. I then started to hear the voices of the two doctors I trusted who kept telling me that my issue was of weight control more than the blood. I even had a few doctors in my city, who wouldn't touch me at all because of the high risk, and not being a surgical candidate for a hysterectomy at that time.

I was all alone at home dealing with this issue of blood, but I coped by staying busy and doing the things that brought me joy. You see, I absolutely loved helping others, especially women, be able to heal and bring joy to them. I did this outside of my "real job" by producing wellness weekend retreats for women, providing coaching to those in need, and I also loved cooking, baking and decorating cakes. It was a complete struggle to continue those things I loved, but I did it. On the surface, it brought me happiness and satisfaction, but beneath it all, I literally struggled daily. Here I was hemorrhaging, barely with any energy, in a job that I grew to hate because it was a hostile-working environment. I became too ill to return to travel nursing and the income I had, I knew I couldn't get any better working in a local hospital or medical facility without being a part of an agency. Due to regulations in the industry, I wouldn't have been able to live locally and work through the agencies. Working for a local medical facility would've been a huge pay cut for me and I would've probably had to get two jobs to replace my income. So, needless to say, I felt stuck and started to walk away from nursing because of my experience.

I was filled with so much anger. I was angry and disappointed with the executive nurses for not believing me when I complained of bad treatment. I was angry at co-workers for wanting to pick my brain constantly but not wanting to stand up for me or anyone else when they saw injustices happening. I was pissed off and disappointed with my husband for not being supportive as he promised he would be. He didn't even try to understand what I was going through until his close, female friend went through a similar problem as I did. However, she was completely operable and I still wasn't. It always seemed to me that my husband's main concern was about whether he was getting some sex today or not. He had always only had to be concerned about himself and everything outside of the home. I naturally took care of everything else. So, when I pulled back, he seemed to only be concerned about how he was going to be taken care of- from laundry, to food, to finances, house issues, and sex. So, this made me even more angry and resentful. Our marriage became a strain the more he pulled away and didn't cater to my needs. Many days, as I was at home alone, I felt forgotten about and lonely. I barely got a phone call from my husband and I sure didn't get any pop up visitations to see how I was doing. He was off living his life and doing any and everything he wanted. His line of work would keep him with very late hours, but he always had his phone. He just didn't use it to check on me often at that time. Because of the neglect and anger I felt, I then found an open arm and listening ear, and it wasn't my husband, nor was it God. I found myself leaning on another man for support. Before I knew it, I was preparing to exit my marriage for good, but then my symptoms worsened. There was no more intermittent bleeding or hemorrhaging. It was now continuous.

Can you imagine having a wound that never stops bleeding? Can you imagine having a wound that is so painful and it never heals? Well, that's what I was experiencing. I had close family and friends who had fibroids and as I spoke with them, the majority of them were mute about their experience and their treatment. Things got worse for me and many days I felt that God should've just let me go already. Here I was married to one man and not connected physically, emotionally, or spiritually, then involved with another man who became obsessive, emotionally abusive, and controlling. There were times I actually feared for my life. Keep in mind, I still was working in my Hell-hole, the "real job". This wound I had was humongous and highly toxic! This was a physical, emotional, and spiritual wound needing to be healed. So, you see, this wasn't a job for any man on Earth. This was a straight up God job and I needed him to fix what I messed up ASAP.

While I was in the battle of my life, I kept hearing and reading about the woman with the issue of blood(Mark 5:25-34). I'm gonna be honest. I got so sick and tired of hearing about this story during that time. I said to myself that I already prayed and I believe I will be healed, but honestly, I really didn't deep down inside. I actually was feeling neglected by God. Truth is, I left him for a bit and didn't realize it. I still believed in God and praised him. I also prayed, but I abandoned the relationship. So, I basically was doing drive-by visitations with Jesus. Why? Well, I knew I wasn't doing what I was supposed to in his eyes. I often wondered if I was being punished for everything. Then, one day I finally saw the light. Here we went revisiting that woman again with the crazy faith in God. There was a reason he kept bringing me to that scripture. I finally paid attention. This woman had suffered enough for well over a decade and she decided enough was enough. She knew that Jesus was her doctor and he was the one to heal her. She, like me, had tried everything else. My issue of blood was deeply rooted.

Although researchers haven't found exactly the root cause of fibroids, God has shown me that it is definitely related to deeply rooted anger, resentment, bitterness, and hatred. He started showing me patterns like during periods where I was most angry, stressed, and just numb in feelings, I hemorrhaged more than ever. When I was most relaxed and without stress, I barely bled or even cramped. He also showed me the more I pulled away from him, the worse my situation became. He showed me that I needed to get rid of the toxicities if I wanted healing and come on back to him- and trust him. So, I did just that. I submitted to God and repented.

I immediately ended the extramarital affair I had and explained to him I needed to be with my husband. Well, he didn't take that well and things got a bit ugly, but God protected me as he promised. I then still needed relief from my "real job" , and God gave me relief from there as well. I was in my office one day burning up at the job stress daily and feeling like I literally had to suit up for battle daily just to go and care for others. I was talking with God and explained that he needed to do something or I was going to hurt somebody. I was immediately reminded that I was supposed to be gone already since two years ago! So, I was at the computer and immediately opened my email and typed a one-sentence, two-week resignation and pressed send. It felt, at that moment, as if I had been constipated for years and finally had relief. The amount of peace and joy that overcame me was so amazing! God is so strategic! Do you know that by my act of obedience, God made it so I only had to work two and a half more days from the time of my typing that resignation email. It was around the fourth of July holiday, plus I already had a doctor's appointment and a vacation day scheduled from weeks prior to that date. God told me that everything he wanted me to do was already within me and I needed to build a better relationship with my husband and lean on him like never before. Remember, I was already doing the retreats, coaching, and baking and cooking. I just had to learn how to monetize it and make these hobbies all legal businesses.

The two major problems I still had were my husband and my fibroids. We started to repair what was broken. My husband apologized for the neglect, owned up to his inappropriate behaviors outside of our marriage, then we began the counseling process. I started for just myself and then we both began counseling together. He then became a great support to me as I was preparing for surgery and had to travel long distance frequently for medical care. By him becoming more of an active participant in my medical care, he then understood the severity of my medical condition. I started to see a change in him. He became very concerned about me and wanted me to be around, therefore, he finally started to step up and take charge of things at home and in our relationship. You see, all I really had to do was submit to God and be obedient. I then had to learn how to truly forgive my husband and pray for him. That's very hard to do if you are holding anger, bitterness, and resentment to the point where you become numb. Your prayers won't even make it past the ceiling like that. I remember when praying for him was the absolute last thing I would have ever thought about. I just wanted out of the marriage because I was sick and tired of being sick and tired! Now, I've learned the importance of praying for him and I've witnessed the many benefits of it. I pray for him all the time when I see any ill behaviors, or if I see that he is attracting certain folks in his life who don't mean him well, or even praying for him to have continued strengthening to become more of the man, husband, and father that God desires him to be. It works!! However, it works with a clean heart! So, forgiveness is a must before doing this.

Finally, after I released myself from the mental, emotional and spiritual prison I placed myself in, God freed me physically and blessed my body and soul because of my continued obedience. Remember, no doctor would touch me locally, and I've traveled to another state having very little surgical hope as well. I then traveled two and a half hours away frequently every two weeks for a few months to be closely monitored and treated for fibroids and severe anemia. I had no iron, I was very short of breath with minimal exertion, severe swelling, obesity, and I had "numerous lesions" along with a large fibroid and a "massive" fibroid- which they described as the "blood sucker". They were positioned in a way where it was difficult to reach. With all of those issues, I kept going to multiple doctors and surgeons for their opinions because ultimately I wanted to be able to have at least one child. I couldn't do this if I had a hysterectomy. Right? Well, after numerous bad reports, I finally gave in and said I would have the surgery. My last "second opinion", for what felt like the fifteenth time was actually on a Monday- the week of my surgery date, which was a Friday. After I gave in and said "God I'm trusting you because you know the desires of my heart". He then immediately reminded me that he already gave me a child and he was assigned to me and my husband to care for. I was to nurture him and show him the way as if he was my own. I instantly became so full of tears and gratitude. I was so busy worrying about something that God had taken care of a year prior. You see, a year prior to my surgery date, my husband and I became overnight parents. We gained custody of my great nephew and rescued him from an abusive home where DSS was involved. We had been nurturing him, but we thought it was to be temporary until God showed us differently. The situation progressed where we eventually acquired permanent custody and he has never been happier. This was definitely a divine assignment and we couldn't have done the setup any better. So, you see, God gave me and my husband the desires of our heart. This child has the personality of my husband and when you put us all together, it's very hard to convince folks that we did not create him because they swear we look alike. He has common characteristics with us and loves to be with family and friends. So, yes, he has definitely been a blessing- just as we have been to him.

Regarding my surgical intervention, everything went well. I had the chief of surgery, chief anesthesiologist, and I was told I was the biggest case that day. I was also warned that there were no guarantees that I could wake up, however, at that moment, I felt ok whether I did or didn't wake up after surgery. My desires and hopes were taken care of by my provider, God. I had no worries and told the surgeon that God sent me here and you and your team's hands have been blessed to help me heal. I had no worries. I remember seeing an overwhelming amount of peace over my surgeon's face and then he said, "Amen". So, eight hours of surgery later, with a nineteen centimeter uterus removed- which was described as the size of a "bowling ball shaped like a football", I survived! I was healed of something that plagued my body for many years. I was finally free! I had many folks tell me that their fibroids dissolved without surgery, well, mine didn't. My process, just as everyone else's process is very different.

During my process, I had to learn how to heal emotionally, regain my spiritual health, and love deeply again. I had to learn to heal myself and understand my assignment more before helping to heal with my husband and helping him to heal. I learned that I had to endure that process in order to deal with and help heal the many broken women who were called to me. That was my process and honestly, I wouldn't trade it for anything. I learned so much. Here are some of my lessons I'm sharing with you: Trust God and lean not on my own understandings. God will give you the desires of your heart for he knows the plans he has for you, before you were even formed. In order to heal your deepest hurts, you gotta be willing to face them first, then forgive yourself and those who have hurt you the worst. Be careful not to allow folks who are afraid of living their dreams tell you how to live. Surround yourself with folks who are actually living their dreams now and not following the crowd and doing what is most popular. Lastly, remember that we have the power to heal- as God didn't create us to have all of this sickness. We can all do such great work on this Earth if we were obedient and healed. Just imagine what this world would look like with billions of HEALED folks operating in purpose and excellence. Just imagine that!

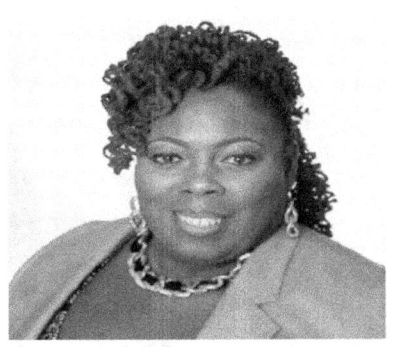

Suprena Hickman-BIO

Suprena was born and raised in beautiful, historic Charleston, SC and loves the coastal region. She currently resides in Wilmington, NC with her husband and is quite involved in her community. She understands what it's like to be "busy" taking care of everyone else besides herself and has successfully crossed that bridge of learning how to make herself a priority in order to better care for others. She has a passion for helping broken women fearlessly pursue their passion and purpose while assisting them to optimal health. She also has great passion for taking care of the caregivers and teaching them to better care for themselves. Her platform to continue this great work is a wellness organization for women called Escape 2 Sisterhood, LLC. Through this organization, she and her partner has been successful in providing wellness retreats for women and social and wellness events to provide an outlet or escape for busy women who are focused on caring for others, advancing their careers, and who tend to place themselves on the back burners. She is also the co-founder of a teen empowerment organization called Girls Rocking In The South, LLC and this is Escape 2 Sisterhood's teen mentoring group. She believes that by helping young teenage girls take care of and respect themselves now then when they become older women, these practices will be incorporated into their daily lives.

Suprena is a Registered Nurse and has worked in many aspects of nursing with over 17 years of experience as a healthcare professional. She has traveled across the country caring for many patients for nearly a decade as a travel nurse and loves assisting in the transformation process. As a nurse/caregiver of many years, Suprena understands what it feels like to sacrifice her personal health and place others' needs before her needs. Now, Suprena is dedicated to helping the caregivers escape! She believes that "the best investment you could ever make is in yourself. The return is priceless"!

Additionally, Suprena is a graduate and proud alum of Norfolk State University where she received her B.S. in Nursing. Also she has her MBA from the University of Phoenix. Suprena is a Certified Integrative Health Coach- trained by Duke Integrative Medicine. She also runs her own bakery business called Sweet Escapes- which was created as an outlet initially from her professional career. Suprena is a member of the following professional organizations: American Nurses Association, National Nurses in Business Association, National Black Nurses Association, North Carolina Nurses Association, & International Coach Federation. Currently, Suprena is a Nurse Entrepreneur focusing on educating and empowering women to invest in their health one escape at a time. Suprena believes in the holistic approach which has been successful over the years with the retreats. As she continues to improve her overall health, she inspires many women to do the same- as it is her passion.

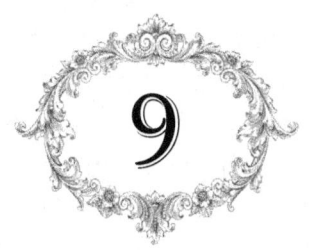

Chapter Nine

SICK, GOING IN CIRLCES

Trisché Duckworth

Anointed, but sick. This is the plight of many believers today. This plight is nothing new to us as Christians, as many people have been suffering silently for years, myself included. Professing that you're stressing seems to be shunned upon, so people maintain the image of having it together when they know full well they're falling apart. It's so hard to not participate in this masquerading, as removing the mask, sometimes, brings forth such judgement and persecution. Funny thing is, those judging, are as sick as, or even sicker, than the ones they judge. So, you have people suffering, hiding their sicknesses from each other, yet manifesting behaviors that would allow anyone to see that something is, ABSOLUTELY, wrong. But let me serve you notice, it's okay to say that you are struggling because it's a part of the process.

I can talk all day about what others may suffer from, but I want to give you a more personal view. Sometimes we need an example so we can relate or even see ourselves in what someone has gone through. I've been in the church ALL my life. I can remember nothing else but going to church, which is why I guess I'm considered what some call a "pew baby" (born into and being reared in the church). The church we were a part of was all I knew, so me searching for GOD outside of that, well that wasn't going to happen. While I love the people of GOD that we fellowshipped with, at that time, some of the things we were taught didn't help me cultivate that true relationship with GOD. See, it's a true relationship with GOD that will sustain you in the midst of the struggle. Living our truth is majorly important to our relationship with GOD. And, if we, really, expect GOD to move in our lives, we must "worship in Spirit and in TRUTH."

So, what does this truth look like? It's not always easy to look at, which is why it's so hard for us to walk in our truth. It means admitting that we see the good, the bad, and the ugly in our lives. It means accepting it for what it is, but always keeping our hearts open for what is to come from the lesson, that might not be pretty. For me, accepting my truth meant going back to the place in my life where I started to believe the lies of the enemy. It meant taking a deeper look past my surface, which is something I knew nothing about. GOD put me in a position where I had to look; I had to see for myself exactly what was keeping me stagnant in life, both spiritually and naturally. I knew there was something different about my life, but I couldn't see past all the hurt and pain. I had suppressed all the pain, so I could survive, but in this moment GOD wasn't having it, HE MADE ME LOOK! HE knew what HE deposited in me and HE wasn't going to let it go to waste. Remember this, what GOD has spoken over you, HE's going to see it through!! It's a done deal!! HE just needs us to participate in HIS plan for our lives.

    Here's where I'll tell you that you can look and still not know what you're looking at, and maintain your place of stagnancy. Seeing is only the first step, but understanding what you see is where you can begin to combat the lies of the enemy. My first look wasn't an easy feat. I didn't want to drum up those old feelings, but it was time. I was serving in the ministry, singing, preaching, teaching, working with the youth, you name it, I was doing it. And all the supposed spiritual folks that I was around, but no one could see that I was working, yet dying on the inside. It was so bad that my serving began to fade away. I was riddled with so much guilt because of the place that I was in, I didn't see that I had anything to offer, ministry wise, so I left building fellowship. There's a reason that I said I left "building fellowship." In my mind, I thought, per what I had been taught, that I was in a backslidden position. I had no clue that GOD was setting me up to deal with what was ailing me, getting ready to propel me further into HIS will for my life.

    As I sat on the outside of "building fellowship" looking in, GOD was still ministering to my heart. HE allowed me to see how I got so busy doing what I thought HE had for me to do, that I moved far away from what HE truly had intended for my life. My robotic worship style, doing things ritualistically, that was no longer going to cut it. HE let me know that it was time to deal with my pain and that my life depended on it. At this time, I was working at a well-known phone company, known as "Ma Bell." So not only was my robotic, ritualistic worship distracting me, the high demands at the telephone company, coupled with a physical ailment I was suffering through, that had me spiraling downhill. Due to health concerns beyond my control, I took a leave of absence from work. Through the process, I also began to see a Therapist and Psychiatrist. All of this was moving so quickly, but I had to go through with it because I knew that GOD was calling for me to begin the journey to my freedom and liberty in HIM.

Counseling/therapy was sooooooooooo hard, but it was sooooooooo necessary. In some African American communities, counseling/therapy is something that isn't a reality and is even frowned upon. Because of the myths surrounding counseling/therapy, I had an extremely hard time when I first started. I couldn't seem to find a therapist that I connected with, which is key to the success of your time working with them. Building that rapport will only allow you to feel more comfortable, which means you'll be more open to share and do the work, whether it's challenging or not. I am, now, a social worker by profession, and to me, building rapport is one of the most important aspects of working with a client during their healing process. Eventually, after two or three therapists, I finally found my match.

Up until this point, I was cruising through life, motivated, but barely making it. She started out by asking me to tell her a bit about myself. This was so hard to do because I didn't, really, know what to say. I'd later learn that I didn't know what to say because I didn't know, THEN, who I was, even though I knew whose I was. Hearing me talk, after just the first session, she could see that I was functioning, yet severely depressed. She didn't know it yet, but I was about to disclose to her that I had been suicidal for a great majority of my life. When I told her, she wasn't shocked. She said, "How you feel about yourself and the things you say let me know that you don't see the value in your life." I was a bit puzzled. I never, really, understood that I didn't see value in my life. The more I thought about it, reflecting back to my life's decisions, all the hurt and brokenness, the unresolved issues, meaningless relationships, terrible, one-sided friendships, even family challenges, I could totally embrace what she spoke.

I didn't see any value in my life, and it started long before I could remember. One thing that I can clearly remember, that shattered my value, was being raped at 13 ½ years old. It was something I didn't see coming. I was an empty child, looking for attention, and guess what, I got it. I met a young man at the park. I had an enormous love for basketball and I guess he picked up on that from seeing me out there. He began to groom me, and of course, I didn't know it. I was just looking to play basketball and chill because I was young and I knew my parents wouldn't tolerate anything else. He told me he was 16 years old, when he was 20. Once I learned how old he was, I ended the very short-term "friendship" (what I thought was a friendship). My dad was a Pastor in one of the strictest denominations on the face of the planet. I knew there'd be no tolerance for any foolishness, which is why I always hid the things I went through.

See I learned early how to wear a mask, which is ultimately living a lie. This lie would alter my life, for a great portion of my life. He raped me and I never uttered a word to anyone, not even my parents. I was scared. It had been drilled in my head that sex was wrong and a sin before GOD. I knew I didn't want it, but in my head, it was the act of sex, and I didn't want to get in trouble. So, for years, I endured that pain inwardly, while reflecting some, not-so-good, behaviors outwardly. I suffered for years and not a soul knew. They saw my not-so-good behaviors, but no one could discern spiritually what had happened, so I got lost in my pain, hiding this vicious violation.

Even though, through the therapy experience, this seemed like something that was terrible to remember, I felt SUPER relieved because I was able to release one thing, of many, that had been plaguing my soul. I knew it was only the beginning and that I would have to continue to dig deep inside, but I felt ready. Remember this, with GOD leading the way, every battle is already won. I began to look, more and more, in the mirror. I wanted to see it all, I wanted to end the pain and finally live free. I was so ambitious, but didn't even understand that I had just scratched the surface, and it was about to get even uglier. When you open the door to believe the enemies lies, you have to travel down the road to replace his lies with GOD's truth, HIS truth about you. That's what made the process hard in the beginning, I had to face all the lies the enemy told me. But the great part was this, canceling out his lies means that the TRUTH OF GOD would heal me and allow me the freedom to walk into my destiny.

Now some have a misconception that you're healed of something and that's it, but baby, let me tell you, it's not that simple. There's sin, then there's the weight of sin, meaning consequences, so as you climb up out of those dead circumstances in your life, you may have to endure some pain, but this pain is different. This pain is one with an expected end. It is one that is turning from hurt into help because all that you've endured wasn't just about you anyways, it was about GOD using you and what you've been through, for HIS Glory, to help somebody else. It's hard not to think selfishly when you're in the midst of the struggle, but I promise you, the other side of it, well it's like the word says, "your latter shall be greater," or even "the sufferings of this world are not worthy to be compared to the GLORY that shall be revealed in us." So part of me sharing today is preparing you to walk out of your moment of pain, into the GLORY. And remember this, no matter what it looks like, as long as you're allowing GOD to work in your life, know that you're on the right track. You may not feel you are where you want to be, but you have to acknowledge that you're not in the same position you were once in. And know that you may still have some issues, but the scriptures also say, "they were healed as they went." So keep it moving to your freedom.

After counseling, which lasted about a year or so, GOD began to move my direction. I started losing everything, and I didn't understand why. I'm ready to celebrate what GOD had done, but clearly GOD was like "AWWWWWWW that's cute, but we got more work to do." I left my job and decided I was moving to the ATL. Notice I said I. You know they say, "if you want to make GOD laugh, tell HIM your plans." I entered a contest to be in a Tyler Perry play and was going to live, what I thought was, my dream. Now remember, this whole dream thing, this walk in your destiny thing, it was all new to me, but I jumped in head first. I packed up my things, went to stay with my big brother, Wilbert, GOD rest his soul, and just knew I was starting my new life in Atlanta. How many know that wherever you go, you're going to be there, meaning whatever your current state is, that is exactly what it will be when you change your geographical location? Long story short, GOD allowed me to be in Atlanta to spend time with my brother before he passed, but it wasn't time for me to move anywhere. So needless to say, my things, that I traveled there with, still in Atlanta to this day, but I still reside in Michigan. See GOD had begun to deal with me, but I wasn't in a place where I could move and start a journey that mentally and spiritually, I wasn't ready for. Really, GOD blocking that move saved me from I don't know what, but it wouldn't have been good!! I am truly thankful to GOD for HIS mercy!!

I came back to Michigan, but I meant business, I still wanted to walk in GOD's designed path for my life and was open to dealing with everything, that I needed to, to get there. GOD was making me deal with my broken relationships with men on this next level. Because of the rape, I was callous and no nonsense towards men, until I met him. He was just as broken as I was and projected his pain on me through the way I allowed him to treat me. Funny thing is, I kept trying to blame him for the pain he was imposing on me. But on this next level, GOD was making me accountable for all my actions. I didn't have to accept what I had allowed in my life. HE allowed me to see that these broken relationships, that I kept subscribing to, were a mere reflection of the deep pain that had been suppressed deep inside of me for years. Even though it was super challenging for years, being accountable kept me moving forward, closer to my destiny. Again, it wasn't easy, but I was seeing, more and more, why it was necessary.

I then started school. I didn't know what I was going for, but I heard the LORD's challenge to go. It came through a dear friend of mine, Darrel Mance. I accepted the challenge and started. I began taking classes for music because I was familiar with that, growing up singing in the church. GOD then guided me right to where I needed to be, social work. I didn't know how I was going to make it through, as I was 36 starting a journey that was completely foreign to me. BUT GOD. I made it through with success. I completed Washtenaw Community

College with an Associate's degree, then on to Eastern Michigan University for a Bachelor's in Social work, then thankfully HE blessed me to obtain a Master's degree in Social work from the University of Southern California. It's funny because I hear folks dismiss people and tell them if they don't have a plan they won't succeed. Well, look here, I didn't have a plan, but through the eyes of CHRIST, I can more and more see GOD's plan and I'm blessed to be walking in it.

Now please don't think that I'm trying to boast, but I want you to understand how GOD can take your thoughts of doom and gloom, bring healing to your life, then allow you to see things HIS way. I learned his way, only through his LOVE, mercy and grace, and for that, every day, I feel extremely grateful. I'm grateful because at a time where I tried to, unconsciously, sabotage GOD's plan, HIS will is being done. I say it's being done because I know that GOD is not done shaping me into HIS masterpiece!! It's already a completed work in HIM, but I'm walking it out, as we pray all the time, "thy kingdom come, thy will be done, on Earth, as it is in Heaven." We are how HIS will is accomplished on this Earth, so HE needs us to move past our pain and into our destiny, which is serving GOD and HIS people in the way that HE has ordained. We all have different paths, but we're similar because we all have a destiny. It is our differences that bind us together, which equates to being a "body jointly fit." Everybody has their place. I found mine and am walking towards my full potential in HIM. And really, we will only arrive at our full potential when there's no more work to do. Then and only then will we have arrived. Until then, we live to learn and grow another day, to fulfill HIS plan in the Earth.

What steps are you taking or have already taken towards your destiny? Whether you must crawl, limp, walk, scoot, whatever, just keep moving. Don't move more into your own mind, but access the mind of CHRIST, move into Heavenly places, as that is where you will find out who you are and how to execute GOD's plan. That is where you can begin to see how you're anointed, yet sick. And trust, that's no death sentence. As a matter of fact, once you realize you are sick, you can begin allowing GOD to show you how to become healed and whole. You owe it to yourself to live the best life that GOD has for you on this Earth, but more importantly you owe it to those that GOD has attached to you, so they can see the GLORY of the LORD in their own lives. People are broken and hurting, they're waiting for a true touch. It's up to us, as the scripture also says, "we overcome by the blood of the Lamb and the word of our testimony." The world is waiting to hear all about your freedom journey. They want to see the blueprint, so they can begin to walk in freedom as well. You may be anointed and sick, but freedom is yours today.

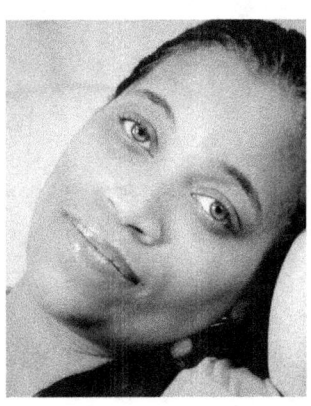

Trische' Duckworth

By profession she is a social worker, who graduated with her Master's Degree in December 2014. She loves to build connections within the community, as well as building bridges between the community and agencies that can offer help to community members in times of distress. Her greatest passion is helping people become who they are destined to be. February 2018, she founded "Survivors Speak", which is a platform that allows people to express what they have or are surviving, in their own creative way. She is committed to sounding the alarm and letting people know that they can make it through any circumstance with the help of GOD. She wants to let the world know that nothing she accomplished is of her own design, rather it's only by HIS. HIS love saved her life, literally, and now she wants to help others see HIS love as well. She also has a street ministry, that she's very passionate about, but still fellowships with a local assembly.

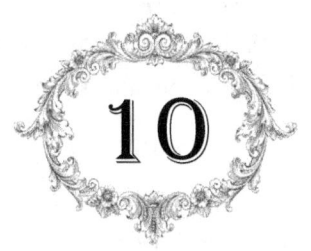

Chapter Ten

EVEN IN THE MIDST

Michelle Tutt

Even in the midst...

Growing up I never saw the hand of GOD. In other words, I saw nothing that I could attribute to GOD, only man. With that said, I didn't have much faith. In fact, I didn't think anyone had much faith. I heard people talk the talk, but I didn't see it manifested in their daily lives. I didn't see them use the wisdom that they read about on Sunday. I didn't see them apply the principles that the Bible spoke of. So, it just boiled down to a ritual or religious practice that allowed them to check a box that said I've done what is expected of me as a Christian (or so they thought). It wasn't until later in life that I received the baptism of the Holy Spirit, that I got an unquenchable desire to learn the things of GOD. This is when my faith began to build. I share this as a prelude to my story because this is how my healing journey began. Up to this time I had never seen anyone divinely healed, or any other kind of miracle for that matter.

My first encounter – It's a miracle!

I had a back problem for 18 years. I reinjured it somewhere along the way and I was diagnosed with a herniated disc. The doctor advised me to have surgery. However, I declined and attempted to use exercises and home remedies. Nothing worked, and I just continued to suffer with debilitating pain. In the meantime, I found a new church where I began to grow by leaps and bounds. My faith was building, and I began to believe God to the point of if He told me I was going to fly around the room... well I would just get ready. So, I was at a Friday night service at my church. My pastor, Pastor John Cherry Sr., said he felt the Holy Spirit leading him not to teach but to have a healing service. So, he proceeded to briefly explain the importance of faith in healing. When he was done, he instructed us on how he wanted us to come up front and that he and Mrs. Cherry were going to lay hands on everyone who wanted healing. I thought, "Great! I need healing." I had just taken 4 pain pills before service started. So, I got in line where Mrs. Cherry was. Now the entire time people were walking around having hands laid on them, he was praying.

This took some time because there were hundreds of people in line. Well I went home moved by the whole service but unaware anything had happened to me. Well the next morning I woke up on my back. You might think that's no big deal. Well for someone who had not been able to lay on their back without experiencing pain.....this was a big deal. What I realized at that moment was, I had been healed. Hallelujah! I got up jumping for joy. That Saturday I put my healing to the test. My yard is 2 acres and even though I had not been able to do yard work, I worked all day. I was bending, carrying tools, digging and pulling tree limbs across the yard. I was healed!!! That was 1996 and I never looked back. I truly believe faith was the key.

A few years later......change on the horizon!

We decided as a family to go on a vacation with the grandkids to Disney World for Thanksgiving. We all drove together in my big suburban. On the way back, my husband and I sat in the back and let my son-in-law drive. I know my legs were cramped but I didn't think much about it. After returning home and getting back to work, I was working late as usual. Actually, it was very late, and I had been sitting at my desk for several hours. When I got up I was short of breath. I thought, that's strange I haven't been doing anything but sitting. I went to the bathroom and then went home. Well that night it kept getting worse and worse. So, I called my HMO. Then they told me to call the office first thing in the morning. Well it was so bad that I thought.... Call?? I'm not calling. I'm going to be there when they open. Well I sat up all night because I was afraid to lay down. So early that morning I headed to Kaiser. It was an hour drive. Well about 45 minutes into the drive this strange feeling came over me and I thought I might be dying. I called and told them I was going straight to the hospital. They told me which one to go to, but I told them I was going to the closest one I could get to. Once there, they thought I was having a heart attack. But after a battery of tests, they discovered I had multiple blood clots in both lungs. I asked how many, but they never answered. I figured they didn't want to scare me with the truth. Well, I was admitted right away. When I got in the room, a nurse came in and said, "You're not supposed to be here!" Meaning she didn't understand how I was still alive. I replied, "Well my Father had something to say about that!" And the thing that I found most amazing was that, as I lay in the hospital having faced near extinction, God was using me to speak into the lives of people who worked in that hospital. In particular, a German nurse who worked at night used to come and sit by my bed and listen to me speak of the goodness of the Lord. I began to believe that the reason that I was there wasn't about me at all.

Through these ordeals I was learning that GOD can defy any rules or logic that man can come up with. GOD is sovereign. If He wants to heal you He can. And I believe your faith has a lot to do with it. Can He heal you if you don't believe? Absolutely. He's sovereign, meaning He can do whatever He wants. However, for the most part, I believe our faith plays a critical part. James 1:6 tells us, "But when you ask, you must believe and not doubt, because the one who doubts is like a wave of the sea, blown and tossed by the wind." And Matthew 21:22 says: "You can pray for anything, and if you have faith, you will receive it." However, remember this, saying you believe because you think it and believing it in your heart and speaking it are two different things. Faith is key in having our prayers answered. Believe it and declare it! Are you speaking faith or doubt and unbelief? Sometimes you may have to keep speaking it until you can believe it. Put a guard on your tongue. Speak only words of faith and watch blessings manifest in your life.

By this point in my life, I saw not only my miracles but many others in the life of my church and pastor. This was so new to me and I was loving it. It gave credence to the Christian life that

I had read about but not seen before. Shortly after my second illness God started to do something very different in my life. He began to use me to bring healing to others. I used to think I wanted to be a nurse. As the years went by I realized I really didn't want to be a nurse. So, what was this pull I was feeling? One morning while I was getting ready for work, I was standing in the bathroom mirror, and the Lord said, "Bind up the wounds." At the time I was planning a women's retreat, so I thought He was giving me the theme. But what I later came to realize was that He was giving me a mandate for my life. This was to be my charge or commission in life. God anointed me to be a vessel of healing. I didn't fully understand this at first, but I just allowed God to slow walk me into it. My primary gift is in emotional healing, although He uses me from time to time in physical healing as well. And many times, He uses me to heal someone else when I myself am going through sickness or great trials.

Sometimes God will sit you down, so you will have time to listen and learn what He wants to teach you. I know that was the case for me. I felt God kept nudging me, but I didn't have time. You know how we do. We act as though we don't hear him. Well, just keep ignoring him. He has a way of getting your attention. Afterward, you will have wished you listened. During the months that I could not work I had plenty of time to ponder on what it was God was trying to say to me. Before this illness I was working 10-12 hours a day in my insurance business. However, when I was unable to work I had a long talk with God. The conversation resulted in me making a commitment to him to give him the time and attention he desired. So, I made a decision to sell my insurance agency and once I was well, I opened a Christian bookstore. Well this was the beginning of major transformation for me. God began to move in miraculous ways. I began to have the time to study his word and pray. I had a room dedicated to prayer. I used to walk the store daily and pray. People started coming in asking for prayer. People were coming in and trusting me with their traumatic life experiences that they had never shared with anyone. This set the stage for emotional healing. He even sent me a friend who had years of experience ministering to hurting women, and she told me she believed God wanted her to teach me what she knew. And as I write this, I remember my need for emotional healing because I had just gone through a traumatic divorce. I wondered why God would choose me to help others heal while I was still in the healing process myself. Isn't it amazing how God works? He uses things that makes no sense to bring healing. What a mighty God we serve!

Well, let me tell you about this prayer room and how God moved mightily through it. It started out as an apartment over the bookstore. There was a tenant in there who was very much behind in rent. After trying to work with him, to no avail, I had to ask him to leave. Well after he moved out, I was anxious to finally get some money, but God told me not to rent it out. With hesitation I said, "Okay Lord. You know I need the money, but nonetheless, if you say don't rent it I won't rent it." So, I didn't rent it out. Well month after month kept passing by and God had not said another word as to what I was supposed to do with it. After many months, my prayer partner and I just decided to start painting and getting it together. Wow! Wow! As soon as we started to move God started to speak. This was a priceless lesson for me. I learned that it takes action on our part to activate the blessings of God. Ooops... there it is! Faith is action. We sit and wait on God but God is waiting on us. Once

I started to move He started to send supplies and people to do everything needed to get this space ready. The mission was in full swing.

During this time God was also preparing me to become a minister. I didn't know it at the time but by having a Christian bookstore, I was being afforded the time to study God's word and he supplied me with all the resources I needed right at my fingertips. I used to say, "God I think you gave me this bookstore just for me." As I was growing and learning the Holy Spirit was steadily moving. I had been on a buying trip to the New York Gift Show and my shipments had started to come in. I was in the bookstore surrounded by boxes when all of a sudden I heard..... "Be instant in season and out of season." This startled me. I was thinking to myself, "What is that supposed to mean?" Well, this kept bugging me, so I called a pastor friend of mine and she told me that was the call to preach. "WHAT??? You've got to be kidding!!!" Well, as it turns out, this was what God was telling me to do. So, I eventually accepted it and moved forward. Actually, I didn't move forward but He moved me forward. God has His way of making things happen. Long story short, the day came for my initial sermon. Afterward, we went out to eat at a local buffet. This man walks up to me as I was returning to my table and asks me if I knew of anyone who needed some pews. I thought that was an odd question to just walk up and ask someone, but I kindly said no. Well, remember that prayer room?

The next day I was thinking about what he said, and I remembered that we were in need of seating for the prayer room. What was I thinking about? So, I got in my vehicle and drove down to where this man's business was. He initially made it sound as if he was giving the pews away but when I got there it turned out he wanted to sell them. They were some very old pews that were left in an old church. Well, after he found out what I wanted them for he told me I could have as many as I wanted, along with anything else I saw that I needed. Well look at GOD!!

GOD really wanted this prayer room and He was making sure that I had everything I needed. He sent someone to paint it for free. He had someone donate a rug. He sent me help to do some of the work, and he gave me strength to sand the hardwood floors. One of the instructions God gave me for this prayer room was to assist people in receiving the baptism of the Holy Spirit. I learned through my own experience that this is critical if we are to walk in the power of God. It wasn't until after I had this experience that I had any life altering or miraculous occurrences in my life. Even though up to this point I had never seen any miracles, once I received the baptism of the Holy Spirit I began to experience miracle after miracle. So enlightening others about it so that they may receive it became a passion for me. I remember one lady received it, but she had no recollection that she had received it or that she had spoken in tongues. All she remembered was that it felt like her tongue split in two. That was amazing because I had never heard anyone describe having that experience that way. Friday night prayer became a very much anticipated event. And the amazing thing is that I spent all of my life in church and had never heard of the baptism of the Holy Spirit and I never knew how to pray. If someone had asked me to stand up and pray I would have probably passed out. We can never know how the anointing of God will change our lives. We just have to be ready to roll with it.

Now during this next season, my health was stable, but I went through a horrific divorce. This period was one of the worst times of my life as far as trials, struggles and satanic attacks. But the most amazing thing is, it was also one of the most fulfilling times of my life also. You see no matter what you go through, I learned that we can still have the joy of the Lord. It truly is our strength! During this time God was giving me direction and instruction in my dreams. He was performing miracles on a regular basis.....all while Satan was kicking up his heels. God seemed to be answering prayer as fast as we could ask. We serve such an amazing God!

Well, the next part of my story continues when a holy ghost filled woman who had converted from Mormonism came into my store. She fell in love with the bookstore and started to come by almost daily. She eventually started volunteering and then became employed there. We would spend time in the store daily praying. She came to the area originally because she had a love one who was incarcerated there. In the past I felt that GOD had been trying to lead me into prison ministry but I kind of averted it. Well now the issue was front and center because during our conversations we would discuss the issues her love one was facing. Well as it turned out, GOD forced my hand and got me involved in prison ministry. The first day I went into the prison, GOD brought back a vison He gave me 20 years prior to me going into the prison. I never knew what it meant until then. The fear then left me and I knew I was anointed for that task. From then on it became a joy. The wisdom of GOD is truly foolishness to man. There was no way I would have ever believed that the things I was doing would give me so much joy. GOD is just amazing. I would have never thought that his desires would lead to the desires of my heart.

It was the most fulfilling experience I'd ever had, but when I went I had no clue what I was going to do. I was just being obedient.

I spent the next 10 years going into the prison on a weekly basis mentoring, teaching, assisting with plays, preaching and occasionally filling in as chaplain. I was fulfilling my God given assignment. During this time my mother became sick with dementia. As she got progressively worse I started missing time from the bookstore. I eventually had to close it altogether. Even with all the changes, I kept my commitment to prison ministry. I was the only child left so there was no other alternative but for me to take care of my mother. She spent so much time taking care of everyone else I could not see putting her in a nursing home. Even amidst financial ruin I stood by my mother. Her disease continued to progress until she passed away. During my time of caring for her I was neglecting myself. If I could pass along any words of encouragement today it would be never neglect self-care. Don't put off routine check-ups. They are so important, especially as you get older.

A couple of years passed after my mother's passing and I started to experience problems with constipation. I have had constipation issues ever since I can remember so I didn't think too much of it at first. Then my problems started to get worse, but I never went to see about it. Finally, about the time that I thought I really need to get to a doctor to get checked out, I woke up one morning in such pain it was unbearable. Off to the emergency room I went. Well at first, they thought I had diverticulitis. They sent me off to another hospital to have some procedure done. Well after a few weeks of checking, I was diagnosed with stage 3 colon cancer. Well Lord, here we go again. I had been through sickness with the Lord before and

I knew He'd be with me just like He had before. I had said before that if I ever got cancer that I would go with a natural treatment, however, when dealing with the need to move quickly to start treatment and the horror of trying to get your health insurance to approve an alternative treatment, I paused. I prayed about it and GOD gave me peace about working with the doctor I had and going through the conventional treatment and that He would be with me through this process.

So that's what I did. I went through chemotherapy, radiation and then chemotherapy again. That was almost a year ago and I have one treatment left. GOD has been amazing. They gave me all this nausea medication and I never got nauseated. My hair never came out. My energy stayed pretty high. I was able to work in my yard every day. I never lost weight and the doctors were amazed at that. In fact, I gained weight (now that didn't make me very happy). Nevertheless, GOD has kept me throughout this whole process and now that I'm wrapping this season up, He's ready to move me on to a new season of fruitfulness.

If there was anything that I wanted to leave with you it's this. Even as you go through the storms of life, and there will be storms, always look for the silver lining in that cloud. Trust that GOD will be your bridge over troubled water. In every trial there is a door of opportunity. Look for it. There is always a lesson to take forward. Ask the Lord, "What is it that I'm supposed to learn from this?" If we take our minds off of the inconvenience, and focus on the lesson, we may find ourselves coming out of these trials sooner.

Just remember, if GOD has anointed you for a purpose, and you become sick, it will not prevent GOD from fulfilling his purpose in you. You just stay focused on completing what GOD has prepared you to do. He'll take care of the sickness. Throughout all of my sicknesses, I refused to focus on or give in to the sickness. I just believe GOD is bigger than any sickness that can come against you. GOD sent you into the earth with a specific purpose. He has anointed you to accomplish that. Do what you have to do in the natural to take care of yourself, but stay focused on whatever GOD is telling you to do. He'll fix your problems. You just give Him the glory that He deserves. Even in the midst your season of sickness, let the GOD of all power, empower you!

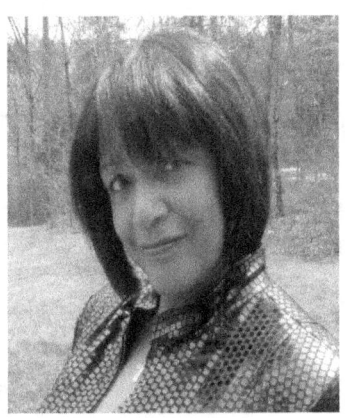

Michelle Tutt-BIO

Michelle Tutt is a woman of God who embraces life and has a passion and dedication to shifting mindsets, facilitating emotional as well as physical healing and being a womb to birth others out into their destiny. She was given a mandate to "bind up the wounds" (Psalm 147:3). She has been self-employed most of her life and is an empowerment coach and founder of New Jerusalem Healing & Restoration Ministries Intl. Her years as a teacher, preacher, mentor and empowerment coach has allowed her to see the devastation of remaining stuck in the same mindset as well as the transformation that is brought about when we allow God to shift our mindset and bring us into a place of blessing.

Michelle also has a passion for the incarcerated. She spent 10 years going into the prisons on a weekly basis with a heart to help them heal the wounds of the past, restore hope and assist them in getting to their original purpose in life. She was highly sought after as a mentor while there.

In this project, she wishes to share with you her journey of healings and what God has taught her through those processes. Our greatest lessons come from our hardest trials. Her desire is for you to stay steadfast and unmovable in your quest for healing, holding on to your faith and not giving in to the naysayers as well as old mindsets of negative thinking.

Be renewed in the spirit of your mind as she takes you through some of her greatest struggles, as she navigated through seasons of sickness and renewal. Be blessed!

If you'd like to contact her she can be reached by email at michelle@empoweredbuilders.com

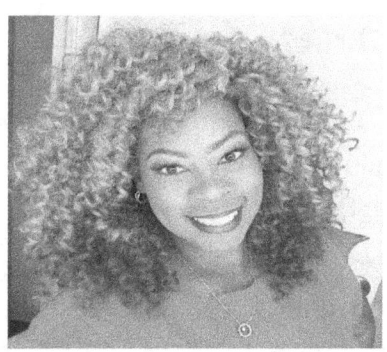

About the Author Dr. Juanita Woodson

Dr. Juanita Woodson is the CEO of Impact Ministries Global and Impact Development Foundation. Dr. Woodson is an apostolic and a prophetic voice with a healing and deliverance ministry who believes in the power of prophecy and prayer. Signs and wonders follow her ministry as well as the testimonies of breakthrough and deliverance by many both nationally and internationally. She is the Founder of Truth Tribe Thursdays also known as T3. T3 is a local ministry that meets on Thursday nights and provides individuals in the Atlanta area a safe place for deliverance, healing, and 5 fold-ministry training. Join Dr. Woodson for the Prophetic Prayer Call held every 2nd and 4th Monday mornings at 9AM EST.

Dr. Woodson has pioneered and founded several non-profit family advocacy agencies that have acquired over $1.5 million in grants since 2008. She is a mompreneur who also built a 6-figure business from home. She is an author, coach, family advocate and inspirational speaker.

Dr. Woodson has a Master's and Doctorate degree in Christian Counseling from Jacksonville Theological Seminary,

Master's Degree studies in Educational Leadership, Bachelor's degree studies in Psychology and History from both Eastern Illinois University and Virginia Commonwealth University. Studies in Antebellum history from the University of the West Indies in Cave Hill, Barbados.

Her mandate is to equip individuals to become everything that God promised they could be and have everything God promised they could have!

www.drjuanitawoodson.com
950 Eagles Landing Pkwy
Suite #722
Stockbridge GA 30281
(678) 614-0016

www.ingramcontent.com/pod-product-compliance
Lightning Source LLC
Chambersburg PA
CBHW071403290426
44108CB00014B/1667